AF892106

OTHER *ESSENTIALS* BOOKS

Essentials on **ADOLESCENT HEALTH FOR NURSING AND HEALTH PROFESSIONALS**: A Care Guide (*Herrman*)

Essentials for the **ADULT-GERONTOLOGY ACUTE CARE NURSE PRACTITIONER** (*Carpenter*)

Essentials for the **ANTEPARTUM AND POSTPARTUM NURSE**: A Nursing Orientation and Care Guide (*Davidson*)

Essentials Workbook for **CARDIAC DYSRHYTHMIAS AND 12-LEAD EKGs** (*Desmarais*)

Essentials for the **CARDIAC SURGERY NURSE**: Caring for Cardiac Surgery Patients, Third Edition (*Hodge*)

Essentials for **CAREER SUCCESS IN NURSING**: Making the Most of Mentoring (*Vance*)

Essentials for the **CATH LAB NURSE**, Second Edition (*McCulloch*)

Essentials for the **CLASSROOM NURSING INSTRUCTOR**: Classroom Teaching (*Yoder-Wise, Kowalski*)

Essentials for the **CLINICAL NURSE LEADER** (*Wilcox, Deerhake*)

Essentials for the **CLINICAL NURSE MANAGER**: Managing a Changing Workplace, Second Edition (*Fry*)

Essentials for the **CLINICAL NURSING INSTRUCTOR**: Clinical Teaching, Third Edition (*Kan, Stabler-Haas*)

Essentials on **COMBATING NURSE BULLYING, INCIVILITY, AND WORKPLACE VIOLENCE**: What Nurses Need to Know (*Ciocco*)

Essentials About **COMPETENCY-BASED EDUCATION IN NURSING**: How to Teach Competency Mastery (*Wittmann-Price, Gittings*)

Essentials for the **CRITICAL CARE NURSE**, Second Edition (*Hewett*)

Essentials About **CURRICULUM DEVELOPMENT IN NURSING**: How to Develop and Evaluate Educational Programs, Second Edition (*McCoy, Anema*)

Essentials for **DEMENTIA CARE**: What Nurses Need to Know, Second Edition (*Miller*)

Essentials for **DEVELOPING A NURSING ACADEMIC PORTFOLIO**: What You Really Need to Know (*Wittmann-Price*)

Essentials About **DIVERSITY, EQUITY, AND INCLUSION IN NURSING**: Building Competencies for an Antiracism Practice (*Davis*)

Essentials for **DNP ROLE DEVELOPMENT**: A Career Navigation Guide (*Menonna-Quinn, Tortorella Genova*)

Essentials About **EKGs FOR NURSES**: The Rules of Identifying EKGs (*Landrum*)

Essentials for the **ER NURSE**: Guide to a Successful Emergency Department Orientation, Fourth Edition (*Buettner*)

Essentials for **EVIDENCE-BASED PRACTICE IN NURSING**: Third Edition (*Godshall*)

Essentials for the **FAITH COMMUNITY NURSE**: Implementing FCN/Parish Nursing (*Hickman*)

Essentials About **FORENSIC NURSING**: What You Need to Know (*Scannell*)

Essentials on **GENETICS AND GENOMICS FOR NURSES**: Practical Applications (*Subasic*)

Essentials for the **GERONTOLOGY NURSE**: A Nursing Care Guide (*Eliopoulos*)

Essentials About **GI AND LIVER DISEASES FOR NURSES**: What APRNs Need to Know (*Chaney*)

Essentials About the **GYNECOLOGICAL EXAM**: A Professional Guide for NPs, PAs, and Midwives, Second Edition (*Secor, Fantasia*)

Essentials in **HEALTH INFORMATICS FOR NURSES** (*Hardy*)

Essentials for **HEALTH PROMOTION IN NURSING**: Promoting Wellness (*Miller*)

Essentials for Nurses About **HOME IN FUSION THERAPY**: The Expert's Best Practice Guide (*Gorski*)

Essentials for the **HOSPICE NURSE**: A Concise Guide to End-of-Life Care, Second Edition (*Wright*)

Essentials about **LGBTQ+ CARE FOR NURSES** (*Traister*)

Essentials for the **LONG-TERM CARE NURSE**: What Nursing Home and Assisted Living Nurses Need to Know (*Eliopoulos*)

Essentials to **LOVING YOUR RESEARCH PROJECT**: A Stress-Free Guide for Novice Researchers in Nursing and Healthcare (*Marshall*)

Essentials for **MAKING THE MOST OF YOUR CAREER IN NURSING** (*Redulla*)

Essentials for **MANAGING PATIENTS WITH APSYCHIATRIC DISORDER**: What RNs, NPs, and New Psych Nurses Need to Know (*Marshall*)

Essentials About **MEDICAL CANNABIS AND OPIOIDS**: Minimizing Opioid Use Through Cannabis (*Smith, Smith*)

Essentials for the **MEDICAL OFFICE NURSE**: What You Really Need to Know (*Richmeier*)

Essentials for the **MEDICAL–SURGICAL NURSE**: Clinical Orientation (*Ciocco*)

Essentials for **MIDWIVES**: Labor & Delivery Orientation, Third Edition (*Groll*)

Essentials for the **OPERATING ROOM NURSE**, Third Edition (*Criscitelli*)

Essentials for **PATIENT SAFETY IN NURSING**: How to Decrease Medical Errors and Improve Patient Outcomes (*Hunt*)

Essentials for **PSYCHOPHARMACOLOGY FOR NURSE PRACTITIONERS** (*Goldin*)

ESSENTIALS About
DIVERSITY, EQUITY, AND INCLUSION IN NURSING

Sandra Davis, PhD, DPM, ACNP-BC, FAANP, is Deputy Director for the National League for Nursing/Walden University College of Nursing Institute for Social Determinants of Health and Social Change. Prior to joining the NLN, Dr. Davis was Associate Professor and Associate Dean for Diversity, Equity, and Inclusion (DEI), at the George Washington University School of Nursing. With over 35 years in faculty, administrative, educator, clinical practice, and leadership roles, her scholarly interests include health inequities, social and structural determinants of health, structural competency, and antiracism.

Internationally, she held DEI discussions at Riverside College in Bacolod, Philippines. Nationally she contributed to the NLN Vision Series titled "A Vision for Integration of the Social Determinants of Health into Nursing Education Curricula" and sits on the National Commission to Address Racism in Nursing. Dr. Davis was Principal Investigator on a Photovoice Project, "The Social Determinants of a Heart Healthy Community," which was exhibited at the Smithsonian National Museum of African American History and Culture. She recently co-published an article in Academic Medicine with Dr. Anne-Marie O'Brien entitled "Let's Talk about Racism: Building Structural Competency in Nursing."

Dr. Davis is a board-certified ACNP and Past President of the NP Association of Washington, DC. She is an AACN/Wharton Executive Leadership Fellow, a Leadership for Academic Nursing Fellow, a Fellow of the American Association of Nurse Practitioners, and an inductee in the Temple University Distinguished Alumni Gallery of Success.

Dr. Davis received a BA from Wellesley College, a BSN from Temple University, an MSN and ACNP certification from the University of Pennsylvania, a DPM from Temple University, and a PhD from Drexel University in Educational Leadership.

Anne-Marie O'Brien, PhD, MA, WHNP-BC, is a nursing professor in the Frances M. Maguire School of Nursing and Health Professions at Gwynedd Mercy University, Gwynedd Valley, Pennsylvania, and a Research Fellow at the Center for Public Policy, Drexel University, Philadelphia, Pennsylvania. She was previously a nurse scientist at Inova Health System and a Clinical Assistant Professor at The George Washington University School of Nursing where she also served as the Director of ABSN Clinical Education. Dr. O'Brien earned her BA in French, her BSN and MSN from the University of Pennsylvania. She earned her MA in French from UCLA. Dr. O'Brien practiced as a women's health nurse practitioner for 9 years in private practice in the field of reproductive endocrinology before going on to earn her PhD in Nursing and Healthcare Innovation with a focus on gerontology from Arizona State University.

Over the last 30 years, she has worked for and with community organizations, academic institutions, and health systems in the belief that we can more effectively address racial and health inequities when we bring together our unique life experiences and expertise. Her clinical practice, research, and teaching have all centered on the social and ecological factors that influence a person's engagement in health promotion and shared decision-making. Dr. O'Brien is also an advocate for social justice and its impact on health disparities, and believes nurses play a crucial role in partnering with communities to make positive change. Dr. O'Brien's research has appeared in The Western Journal of Nursing Research, Nursing Research, Medical Research Archives, and Academic Medicine. Her program of research continues to critically examine institutional and societal power structures and to identify strategies for promoting health equity and social justice.

ESSENTIALS About DIVERSITY, EQUITY, AND INCLUSION IN NURSING

Building Competencies for an Antiracism Practice

Sandra Davis, PhD, DPM, ACNP-BC, FAANP

Anne-Marie O'Brien, PhD, MA, WHNP-BC

SPRINGER PUBLISHING

Springer Publishing Company, LLC
11 West 42nd Street, New York, NY 10036
www.springerpub.com
connect.springerpub.com/

Acquisitions Editor: Rachel X. Landes
Compositor: Transforma

ISBN: 978-0-8261-8452-8

Printed by LSI

The *Essentials* series was published in the United States of America as the *Fast Facts* series.

To our students, colleagues, clients,
and communities with whom we partner
in promoting racial healing and justice.

Contents

Foreword

A wise man once shared that there is a time to plant and a time to uproot what was planted…a time to break down and a time to build up…a time to rip apart and a time to sew together. Indeed, Drs. Davis and O'Brien are publishing *Essentials About Diversity, Equity, and Inclusion in Nursing* at a time when the nursing profession seeks to uproot the remnants of racism, build up the discipline by valuing inclusivity and denouncing racism, and unite diverse voices willing to co-create an antiracist workforce.

During the Tuskegee experiment in 1932, the death of Emmett Till in 1955, and countless other inhumane atrocities, nursing coexisted alongside institutions that endorsed de jure and de facto discrimination and segregation. It is unlikely that any system could have escaped the interlocking power and false doctrine of white supremacy, including nursing, a discipline built on compassion. The profession had to acknowledge that the venomous toxicity of racism had penetrated nursing and created a chasm between the ways the professional values were espoused and operationalized. Until recently, racism operated well beneath a veil of silence that muted discussions on racism. However, the heinous murder of Mr. George Floyd called into question discriminatory beliefs and practices that grew out of the 19th century and exposed the seemingly race-neutral policies that promulgated a century-long homogenous nursing workforce. In 2020, a plethora of nursing organizations across the country sought to not only distance themselves from racism but to disentangle the profession from the roots of injustice and upend discriminatory practices that the discipline once failed to acknowledge.

The authors have responded in a timely fashion to the increasingly diverse number of nurses who seek to educate themselves on meaningful ways to address upstream factors that have resulted in generations of inequities and disparate outcomes in education and healthcare. The book provides compelling evidence that indicts racism as the greatest threat to nursing and emboldens nurses to begin race-related discourse that centers on racism. A brief history reveals how the nursing profession traveled beside legalized discrimination, white supremacy, and racist acts of violence before and beyond the 20th century. Poignant narratives paint a shocking, yet vivid description of discriminatory acts described as microaggressions or slights invisible to the undiscerning eye, albeit potentially greater in significance to the internal mind. Historically racialized individuals will undoubtedly nod in unison with a tearful sigh as they read through the stories and recall similar encounters.

The title of the book should not be erroneously equated to quick approaches to annihilating racism. To be sure, there is no panacea or expedient remedy to stomp out racism. The authors provide evidence-based strategies that move the reader along a continuum that allows for reflective practice and actions as a nurse-citizen. The authors conclude with a list of resources that read like a stepwise approach for the undoing of racism. The book is for novice and expert nurses who seek to gift future providers with a profession prepared to live up to its ideals. I commend the authors for their dynamic collaboration and ability to get this book into the hands of colleagues who want to begin antiracism work if only shown how.

Kenya V. Beard, EdD, AGACNP, CNE, ANEF, FAAN

Foreword

My experiences as a Black female researcher, educator, writer, and administrator have underscored the unique challenges of productive and meaningful discourse on topics of racism, racial justice, health equity, oppression, and power. *Essentials About Diversity, Equity, and Inclusion in Nursing* skillfully illuminates foundational elements of race and racism and highlights leverage within the nursing profession to address subsequent health disparities. Drs. Sandra Davis and Anne-Marie O'Brien equip readers with perspectives and strategies to engage in profound, consequential, and brutally honest conversations about advancing health equity and antiracist practices. The nursing profession has long needed to extend its focus beyond cultural competency and diversity. We must obtain critical self-awareness about racial inequities associated with social structures, automatic and implicit biases, patterns of behaviors, and decision-making that embeds racism into the nursing profession. Dr. Davis, a leader and pioneering scholar in diversity, equity, and inclusion, and Dr. O'Brien, a nurse scientist committed to advancing health equity and building structural competency in nursing, are both well positioned to present strategies to incorporate diversity, equity, inclusion, belonging, and antiracism into nursing practice. *Essentials About Diversity, Equity, and Inclusion in Nursing* is a rallying call to the nursing profession, promoting awareness, continued learning, and individual/collective efforts to restructure systems of oppression that shape how people perceive and navigate the world.

Of great importance, Drs. Davis and O'Brien explicitly highlight that we cannot disconnect the past from the present. James Baldwin (1966) notes that "*[History] does not refer merely, or even principally, to the past. On the contrary, the great force of history comes from the fact that we carry it within us, are unconsciously controlled by it in many ways, and history is literally present in all that we do. It could scarcely be otherwise, since it is to history that we owe our frames of reference, our identities, and our aspirations* (p.174)." The authors hold a mirror up, enabling readers to meet the conscious and subconscious drivers of their core convictions and beliefs head-on. They invite readers to dive deeper, presenting relevant Essential Facts, rich scholarly material, case studies, and critical questions for self-reflection.

The authors' incredible work is rooted in the integral role of holism in health/healthcare and the duty to incorporate social justice practice into the nursing profession. Ultimately, they highlight the pivotal role nurses play in uplifting patients' and communities' humanity and provide key tools to facilitate nurses' evolution into high-performing nurse-citizens. As professional nurses, we must embark on and commit to mobilizing collectively to eradicate both structured and interpersonal racism within the healthcare system. Drs. Davis and O'Brien, with great care and keen astuteness, remove cultural blind spots within the nursing profession. They urge nurses to move from ambivalence, ignorance, passivity, rationalization, and/or mere good intention regarding health and racial equity toward a more progressive model of informed, intentional, and proactive nursing practice in the form of resource distribution, policies, practices, and accountability. These advancements will raise the standard of the nursing profession by investing in patient–provider relationships as well as health systems' responsiveness to communities. We have long needed literature like *Essentials About Diversity, Equity, and Inclusion in Nursing*, but the most recent health inequities exacerbated by state-sanctioned violence and disparate COVID-19 morbidity/mortality further necessitate this book. We are in an optimal place and time to trailblaze and demonstrate why nursing is lauded as the most trusted profession. Drs. Davis and O'Brien's *Essentials* is a must-read for all nurses!

Roberta Waite, EdD, PMHCNS-BC, FAAN, ANEF

REFERENCE

Baldwin, J. (1966). Unnameable objects, unspeakable crimes. In Ebony (Ed.), *The White problem in America* (pp. 173–181). Johnson.

Preface

This book was written at a time like no other in our nation's history. With the convergence of *Healthy People's 2030* goals for achieving health equity, eliminating disparities, and improving the health of all groups; *The Future of Nursing's 2020–2030* call for all nurses to recognize their responsibility to address racism; and the creation of the *National Commission on Racism in Nursing* with a membership represented by more than 20 professional nursing organizations, we are now seeing the necessary and long overdue attention to racism as a public health crisis.

Whereas the root causes of heath inequity are complex and can be found in the structural determinants of health that differentially shape the conditions in which people are born, grow, live, work, and age, racial health inequities have remained entrenched over time and are seemingly intractable. Black maternal and infant mortality rates are avoidable, unjust, unacceptable, and indeed constitute a public health crisis. Despite decades of awareness about these inequities, there is finally an urgent call to examine racism as a root cause of these preventable deaths.

There is also a growing emphasis in both academia and clinical practice to examine those institutional policies and practices that contribute to racial inequities. Many health professions' educational programs are also advancing toward an equity and justice lens to equip the current and future workforce with the knowledge, attitudes, and skills to function in an increasingly diverse world and to eliminate the unjust and avoidable inequities in access to care, the delivery of care, and the resultant health disparities that have persisted far too long in this country.

To more effectively address inequities, the World Health Organization recommends that the education of healthcare professions' students on the social determinants of health be framed within a country's sociopolitical context. For the United States of America, this means confronting the contradictions of our country's past (land of the free for some, but not all) in order to understand our present (significant racial inequities in both health and wealth). Race matters in the United States. Since the beginning, race and racism have been a part of this nation's politics and culture. As difficult as it may be, we must acknowledge our country's collective racist history in order to end those cultural norms and policies that perpetuate disparities and inequities.

Thus, as health professions' curricula move away from pedagogies that focus on multicultural approaches for understanding differences and inequities and toward a recognition of the broader impact that both systemic and structural racism have had on inequities in health and life chances, students, educators, practitioners, and administrators are finding it necessary to engage in critical discourse around topics that were once considered taboo. This new critical paradigm shift for talking about inequities involves uncovering its root causes. And yet, the terms and concepts necessary for engaging in this level of critical discourse have many people wondering what does this all mean? While terms such as structural competence, antiracism, White privilege, implicit bias, and microaggressions are now part of our public lexicon and dialogue, what do they mean to the health professional's individual practice and their workplace setting? Increasingly acceptance, avoidance, and/or silence are no longer suitable approaches to dealing with the persistent disparities and inequities in every sector of our society, including income, housing, criminal justice, and education, that impact health and health outcomes.

Regardless of what stage you are in your work toward eliminating disparities, promoting health equity, and fostering a more inclusive society, this book is a valuable resource for educators, students, and clinicians alike. In this book, we define terms, provide the necessary historical context for gaining insight and understanding into why issues of race, racism, power, privilege, and oppression contribute to inequities in health and economic opportunity, and why the needed work toward this change really is *all of ours* to own.

As we commit ourselves to eliminating racism and health inequities in this country, nurses are now poised at the nexus of reluctance and resistance, truth and reconciliation, and healing and transformation. We hope this book helps you and your fellow nursing colleagues in creating the clinical and educational spaces that not only promote inclusion and feelings of belonging, but also foster a true sense of unity in our collective work toward a more just and equitable society.

Acknowledgments

I would like to acknowledge, with sincere gratitude, the unwavering support from my mother, Virginia Davis, and my sister, Deborah Davis; the memory of my father and my brother; the love and joy from my family; the inspiration from friends; and the interest of colleagues. In addition, it is with appreciation and respect that I acknowledge the connectedness of this work to those past and present, known and unknown who have lived, loved; fought, taught; died, cried; rejoiced and risen above silently, collectively, resoundingly for peace, justice, and equity.

–Sandra

I would like to thank my parents, Jerry and Suzanne O'Brien, who taught me the importance of speaking out against injustice and joining causes that promote equal voice and opportunity for all. I also want to thank my husband and research partner, Dr. Robert J. Kane and our two sons, Liam and Aidan. I could not have done this work without their incredible support. Finally, I want to thank my many BIPOC colleagues, friends, and community members who have welcomed me as a partner in the shared work of creating a more just and equitable future for all Americans.

–Anne-Marie

Together, we would like to acknowledge and thank our amazing editorial team at Springer Publishing: Rachel Landes, Hannah Hicks, and Elizabeth Nieginski. We are grateful for their expert guidance on this book.

Finally, we would like to deviate from convention and acknowledge not only people, but also the process of working together: seeking, connecting, knowing, being, and becoming while searching for and finding meaning.

–Sandra and Anne-Marie

Introduction

The disproportionate impact of COVID-19, the racial injustices in the United States, and the months of world-wide protests underscore the *outrage and despair* over inequity in this country and the work that must be done to disrupt centuries of structural racism. We are living a pivotal moment in history. Now, like never before, America is showing the *willingness* to both discuss and address structural racism.

Colleges and universities, healthcare systems, nonprofit and for-profit organizations, and government agencies alike are examining their commitment not only to diversity, equity, and inclusion, but also to making explicit their commitment to antiracism. At the same time, students are demanding a curriculum that prepares them to close the gap on racism, bias, discrimination, and inequity and to ultimately create a more just and equitable society for all.

Similarly, *The Future of Nursing 2020–2030* report emphasizes nursing's imperative to acknowledge, confront, and dismantle systems of structural racism, including racism in nursing. Indeed, each of us is being called to action to address racism as a root cause of inequities in health and opportunity. In order to develop a workforce prepared to eliminate racism and promote racial equity and opportunity, academic and clinical nurse educators must equip themselves with the knowledge, skills, and attitudes needed to address structural racism and then identify strategies that foster open, respectful dialogue and discovery in their teaching and learning environments. Nursing leaders and administrators will also need to engage fully in this process and support faculty, students, employees, and staff in this work.

Each chapter of our book contains a case study with reflection questions that can be used in teaching and learning environments to promote deeper awareness and understanding of the complex factors that have contributed to persistent racial inequities. At the end of this book, we have curated a multimedia toolkit with up-to-date interactive resources (including music, videos, articles, and podcasts). The toolkit resources can be for individual or group-level reflection, contemplation, dialogue, and growth. Ultimately, we hope this book helps move each of us to engage in deeper, more meaningful, and honest conversations with colleagues about what each of us can do individually and collectively to promote health equity, opportunity, and a sense of belonging for all.

1

Why It Is Important to Talk About Race and Racism

"Race matters."

—Cornel West

As Americans, we are adept at living in a state of contradiction. We live in a racialized society where yes, indeed, race matters. Race is the first thing we see when encountering another person. In fact, we immediately categorize people into racial groups. Yet, we have been socialized not to talk about race and were taught not to talk about race in polite conversation. Moreover, when we do talk about race, discomfort, defensiveness, and frustration often prevail, with comments surfacing such as: get over it, it happened 400 years ago, that's in the past, we had a Black president, I don't see color, or you are too sensitive, *and the conversation shuts down. To eliminate health disparities and achieve health equity we must connect our past to our present and grow comfortable with conversations about race, racism, and racial justice. This chapter helps to move the dialogue from frightening, feared, difficult, and sensitive to necessary, meaningful, and productive.*

After reading this chapter, the reader will be able to:

1. Discuss why it is so difficult to talk about race and racism
2. Explain necessary terms for engaging in conversations about race and racism
3. Describe the importance of discussing race, racism, and the nursing profession

The nursing profession, which has traditionally focused on culture, must begin paying attention to and discovering ways to dialogue about race, racism, and racial justice (Davis & O'Brien, 2020). Cultural competency has been used in nursing education and practice to address health disparities and promote health equity (Davis & O'Brien, 2020; Waite & Nardi, 2021). However, addressing health disparities and promoting health equity must start with an understanding of structural inequities and systems of oppression that started with the founding of our nation (Byrd & Clayton, 2001). Most nursing students and faculty have limited historical knowledge of the legacy of chattel slavery in America (Waite & Nardi, 2021). The right to enslave humans was integrated into the systems and structures of America, including government laws and policies, social interactions, housing, education, and health care (Hammond et al., 2019). Race and racism matter in nursing (Beard & Julion, 2016; Hassouneh, 2006). At the crux of change is understanding how these systems sustain the oppressive practices, stereotyping, health inequities, inferior education, and inadequate access to healthcare that persist today (Hammond et al., 2019).

When talking about race and racism, we cannot disconnect the past from the present. We must acknowledge our history. Further, there is a language for talking about race and racism (Waite & Nardi, 2021). We must learn that language and feel comfortable using it. Nursing faculty and leaders cannot teach and practice what they do not know. (Waite & Nardi, 2017)

Race and Racism Vocabulary

Antiracism: The active process of identifying and eliminating racism by changing systems, organizational structures, policies, practices, and attitudes, so that power is redistributed and shared equitably (National Action Committee International Perspectives: Women and Global Solidarity).

Historical trauma: Originates from the suppression of Black, Indigenous, and People of Color (BIPOC) by racially White populations. Specifically, for Black people, historical trauma is "the collective spiritual, psychological, emotional, and cognitive distress perpetuated intergenerationally deriving from multiple denigrating experiences originating with slavery and continuing with pattern forms of racism and discrimination to the present day" (Waite & Nardi, 2021; Williams-Washington, 2010; Williams-Washington & Mills, 2018, p. 247).

Colonization/colonialism: Some form of invasion, dispossession, and subjugation of a people. Ongoing and legacy colonialism impacts power relations and includes establishing an economic and political power base with the aim of achieving wealth, territory, and dominion of one group over another.

American colonization, manifested through configurations of power, was instrumental in the construction of the concept of race (Waite & Nardi, 2017). It has been used to justify inequitable power relations between settlers and Native Americans as well as persons of African, Hispanic, and Asian descent (Waite & Nardi, 2017).

Racialization: A process of constructing groups founded on physical characteristics that are socially described as significant (Lewis, 2004; Waite & Nardi, 2021). In social systems it involves a hierarchy that produces social relations among the races (Bonilla-Silva, 2001). In addition, it is used when describing Black and Brown racial populations, rendering whiteness invisible, unnamed, and viewed as natural (Waite & Nardi, 2021).

AntiBlack racism or antiblackness: Includes prejudices, attitudes, behaviors, beliefs, practices, stereotyping, discrimination, and/or policies that explicitly or implicitly racialize Black people as inferior to other racial groups, and is rooted in the history and experience of enslavement and its legacy (Waite & Nardi, 2021).

White supremacy: "A political, economic, and cultural system in which whites overwhelmingly control power and material resources" (Ansley, 1989, p. 1024).

Whiteness: The historical and social construction of being white, including social status, privilege, and power linked with being White (Beckles-Raymond, 2020; Waite & Nardi, 2021). Whiteness in America is inherently associated with the enslavement of African people (chattel slavery) and oppressive practices, from European colonization of Indigenous lands in North America to Jim Crow laws, lynching, red-lining, and the continuous racial domination and discrimination of the present (Beckles-Raymond, 2020; Waite & Nardi, 2021).

White privilege: An unearned advantage and the unrecognized benefit of being White (McIntosh, 1989; Waite & Nardi, 2018).

Power: The ability to influence others and impose one's beliefs. It is power and policy that keep racism firmly entrenched in society (Belli, 2020).

Oppression: The systematic subjugation of one social group by a more powerful social group for the social, economic, and political benefit of the more powerful social group (Race Equity Tools, 2020).

Systemic Racism refers to how discriminatory actions against racialized groups occur in systems including but not limited to the educational, criminal justice, and healthcare systems (Slater, 2021).

Structural Racism refers to the totality of ways in which societies foster racial discrimination through mutually reinforcing systems of housing, education, employment, earnings, benefits, credit, media, healthcare, and criminal justice. These practices reinforce discriminatory beliefs, values, and distribution of resources (Bailey et al., 2017, p. 1453).

Levels of Racism

The classic allegory of the Gardener's Tale provides a theoretical framework for understanding racism on three levels: (1) institutionalized, (2) personally mediated, and (3) internalized (Jones, 2000).

Institutionalized: The structures, policies, practices, and values that result in differential access to goods, services, and opportunities by race.

Personally mediated: Differential assumptions about another person's abilities, motives and intents based upon race, which is prejudice, and then having differential actions based on those assumptions, which is discrimination.

Internalized: The acceptance of negative messages about one's abilities and intrinsic worth by members of stigmatized races.

It is important to note that structural racism, systemic racism, and institutional racism are often used interchangeably. However, they do differ in terms of describing how racism operates. Institutional racism occurs within and across institutions while systemic and structural racism are broader terms (Institute Staff, 2016).

Why It Is Difficult to Talk About Racism

While we talk broadly about racism as a root cause of health inequities and a barrier to achieving health equity, we cannot ignore the conversation about race and racism specifically in the nursing profession. Both the beginnings and evolution of the nursing profession are rooted in American colonialism (Waite & Nardi, 2017). Foundational knowledge of race and racism as products of colonialism can help us understand that nursing in the United States began with an institutional bias against Blacks (Waite & Nardi, 2017; Whelan, 2015). As evidenced by Blacks making up only 10.8% of chief nursing officers, the marginalization of Black nurses continues to be seen today at every level, particularly in nursing leadership positions (Nardi et al., 2020; Waite & Nardi, 2017; Zippia The Career Expert, 2021).

Despite this history of racism in the nursing profession, the word and topic of racism have been taboo in nursing. There are attributes of nursing that allowed nurses to avoid openly dealing with racism and have created a culture of denial, color-blindness, and aversive racism (Barbee, 1993). Moreover, nursing continues to believe that racism is an individual attribute rather that a deeply ingrained attitude in nursing and in American society (Barbee, 1993; Waite & Nardi, 2017). Nurse leaders must accurately see it as it is—a systemic, enduring structure that influences everything in the United States including professional nursing practice (Barbee, 1993; Waite & Nardi, 2017). Structural changes that work toward racial equity in the nursing profession require constant intentional efforts that include the involvement of individuals and organizations from multiple layers (Nardi et al., 2020).

Essential Facts

- Segregated hospitals and educational systems for White and Black nurses existed well into the 20th century (Barbee, 1993).
- The Nurses Associated Alumnae of the United States and Canada, formed in 1911, refused to include or support nurses of color (Waite & Nardi, 2017).
- Because of the lack of attention, Black nurses formed their own organizations. The first of these was the National Association of Colored Graduate Nurses (NACGN), which was founded in 1908 (Waite & Nardi, 2017).
- The National Black Nurses Association (NBNA) was formed because of racism in nursing (Barbee, 1993).
- The Association of Black Faculty in Schools of Nursing (ABNF) was founded in 1989 because of the difficulties that Black nurses had with publishing in nursing journals (Waite & Nardi, 2017).

Transparency and openness about not only the history but also the persistence of racism and its effects on the nursing profession are necessary in order to control and achieve diversity, equity, inclusion, belonging, and antiracism (Trueman et al., 2011). The broader foundation of American colonialism, which embeds a system of racism and maintains white supremacy, affects everyone in society including nurses who often enter our profession as a calling because they care and want to improve the health of all people (Schroeder & DiAngelo, 2010). "[To] decolonize the nursing profession" will require courage, intentional actions, and an appreciation of the history that set us on this path (Waite & Nardi, 2017, p. 18). Day and Beard (2019) provide nurse educators with a "culturally responsive teaching" framework to facilitate this change. For example, rather than learning about one "dominant" narrative, students are encouraged to share and learn about diverse cultural backgrounds, norms, and ways of thinking (Day & Beard, 2019). Similarly, Valderama-Wallace and Apesoa-Varano (2019) call on academic nursing programs to not only re-imagine how they address the critical issues of culture, health equity, and antioppression, but also how they invest in their diversity, equity, and inclusion initiatives.

Essential Facts

"Racism is a system of structuring opportunity and assigning value based on the social interpretation of how one looks (which is what we call 'race'), that unfairly **disadvantages** some individuals and communities, unfairly **advantages** other individuals and communities, and saps the strength of the whole society through the waste of human resources." (Jones, 2018, p. 231)

This definition of racism by Dr. Camara Phyllis Jones (2018), is a particularly good starting point for a conversation about race because it demonstrates how race, racism, and racial justice are inextricably connected. Moreover, it allows us to see the systemic nature of racism and how, from the very beginning, America was built on systems of power and oppression and inequality. This lens also allows us to take a "no shame, no blame" approach to becoming *equity-minded* and building bridges of understanding and trust. Moreover, it helps us to realize that discussing race, racism, and racial justice is not about trying to decide whether someone is a racist. Talking about race is important because it will allow us to experience our shared humanity. This is going to involve talking and listening to the stories of others and listening and believing how racism exists and operates.

Strategies for Gaining Knowledge and Building Confidence to Have Conversations About Race and Racism

- Increase your knowledge about the history of race and racism in America
- Understand the language of racism
- Get to know people who do not look like you
- Engage in self-reflection
- Listen to the stories of others

Safe and Brave Spaces

Establishing ground rules or guidelines for engaging in dialogues about race and racism helps to create a reassuring learning environment that invites honesty, sensitivity, and respect (Arao & Clemens, 2013). Facilitators of conversations about race and racism usually present the rules and ask for agreement. Some facilitators may use a hybrid approach where they present a couple of rules and then ask the participants to come up with what they see as important to creating a safe environment for dialogue (Arao & Clemens, 2013). These environments are often referred to as *safe spaces*. Common ground rules for safe spaces generally include (a) agree to disagree, (b) don't take things personally, (c) challenge by choice, (d) show respect, and (e) no attacks (Arao & Clemens, 2013).

Brave spaces focus more on the challenges inherent in conversations about race and racism among diverse participants (Arao & Clemens, 2013). Participants are encouraged to be brave in exploring content that pushes them to the edge of their comfort zones (Arao & Clemens, 2013). Brave spaces help to disrupt and decenter dominant narratives in which knowledge flows one way; for example, from teacher to student (Arao & Clemens, 2013).

Acosta and Ackerman-Barger (2017) suggest that health professionals look to other disciplines for tools and strategies for discussing race and racism. They recommend Glen Singleton's (2014) protocol for having courageous conversations about race and racism. Singleton (2014, p. 70 and pp. 87–214) recommends four agreements and six conditions for providing a safe, open, and honest space for discussions about race and racism.

Singleton's Four Agreements

1. Stay engaged
2. Experience discomfort
3. Speak your truth
4. Expect and accept a lack of closure

Singleton's Six Conditions:

1. "Establish a racial context that is personal, local, and immediate"
2. "Isolate race while acknowledging the broader scope of diversity"
3. "Develop an understanding of race as a social/political construction of knowledge, and engage multiple racial perspectives to surface critical understanding"
4. "Monitor the parameters of the conversation by being explicit and intentional"
5. "Establish agreement around a contemporary working definition of race allowing for a more effective dialogue about race, racism, and racial disparities"
6. "Examine the presence and role of Whiteness and its impact on the conversation" (Singleton, 2014, pp. 81–241)

We need to understand that in this country there are people just like you who are as kind, funny, generous, smart, and hardworking, but live in different circumstances from yours (Kaiser Permanente, 2016). When we are willing to step outside of our own experiences to listen, learn, dialogue, and engage with others, we move toward experiencing our common humanity (Kaiser Permanente, 2016). Once we engage and hear the stories of others and how racism shapes those stories, we then believe the stories of others (Kaiser Permanente, 2016).

Talking about race and racism is so important because only then will we be moved to join in the stories of others to dismantle this system that is adversely impacting us all (Kaiser Permanente, 2016).

CASE STUDY 1.1

Lisa is a second year nursing student taking a community health course. During one of the last days of class, students were discussing social determinants of health and their community heath projects. One student talked about Black Lives Matter Plaza in Washington, D.C. as it was part of her community assessment. Lisa asked to speak to the professor after class. She said that she was afraid to speak up in class but really did not understand why so much of class time was spent talking about Black Lives Matter because that did not have anything to do with social determinants of health. Furthermore, she said that open discussions about race and racism like that make her feel very uncomfortable, are too political, and should not be discussed in the classroom.

Case Study Questions

1. How would you respond to Lisa's concerns?
2. What strategies or approaches might you use to increase students' willingness to engage in class discussions about race and racism? Ibrahim (n.d.) created a visual personal journey and accountability model for engaging in conversations about racism and building an antiracist practice.

REFERENCES

Acosta, D., & Ackerman-Barger, K. (2017). Breaking the silence: Time to talk about race and racism. *Academic Medicine*, *92*(3), 285–288.

Ansley, F. L. (1989). Stirring the ashes: Race class and the future of civil rights scholarship. *Cornell Law Review*, *74*, 993–1077.

Arao, B., & Clemens, K. (2013). From safe to brave spaces. Retrieved on 29 August, 2021, from https://www.gvsu.edu/cms4/asset/843249C9-B1E5-BD47-A25EDBC68363B726/from-safe-spaces-to-brave-spaces.pdf

Bailey, Z. D., Krieger, N., Agenor, M., Graves, J., Linos, N., & Bassett, M. T. (2017). Structural racism and health inequities in the USA: Evidence and interventions. *Lancet*, *389*(10077), 1453–1463.

Barbee, E. L. (1993). Racism in nursing. *Medical Anthropology Quarterly*, *7*(4), 346–362.

Beard, K. V., & Julion, W. (2016). Does race still matter in nursing? The narratives of African-American nursing faculty members. *Nursing Outlook*, *64*, 583–596.

Beckles-Raymond, G. (2020). Implicit bias, white ignorance, and bad faith: The problem of whiteness and anti-black racism. *Journal of Applied Philosophy*, *37*, 169–189. https://doi.org/10.1111/japp.12385

Belli, B. (2020). Kendi: Racism is about power and policy, not people. *Yale News*, December 7, 2020. https://news.yale.edu/2020/12/07/kendi-racism-about-power-and-policy-not-people

Bonilla-Silva, E. (2001). *White supremacy & racism in the Post-Civil Rights Era*. Lynne Rienner Publishers.

Byrd, W. M., & Clayton, L. A. (2001). Race, medicine, and health care in the United States: A historical survey. *Journal of the National Medical Association*, *93*(3), 11S–33S.

Davis, S., & O'Brien, A.-M. (2020). Let's talk about race: Building structural competency in nursing. *Academic Medicine*, *95*(12S), S58–S65. https://doi.org/10.1097/acm.0000000000003688

Day, L., & Beard, K. V. (2019). Meaningful inclusion of diverse voices: The case for culturally responsive teaching in nursing education. *Journal of Professional Nursing, 35*(4), 277–281.

Hammond, J. H., Massey, A. K., & Garza, M. (2019). African-American inequality in the United States. Harvard Business School. https://services.hbsp.harvard.edu/api/courses/733124/items/620046-PDF-ENG/sclinks/1342e4a633014f425f504af2a2d00b86

Hassouneh, D. (2006). Anti-racist pedagogy: Challenges faced by faculty of color in predominantly white schools of nursing. *Journal of Nursing Education, 45*(7), 255.

Ibrahim, A. M. (n.d). A surgeon's journey through research and design. https://www.surgeryredesign.com/current

Institute Staff. (2016, July 11). Terms you should know to better understand structural racism. Aspen Institute. Racial Equity. https://www.aspeninstitute.org/blog-posts/structural-racism-definition/

Jones, C. P. (2000). Levels of racism: A theoretical framework and a gardener's tale. *American Journal of Public Health, 90*(8), 1212–1215.

Jones, C. P. (2018). Toward the science and practice of anti-rasicm: Launching a national campaign against racism. *Ethnicity and Disease, 28*(Suppl 1), 231–234

Jones, C. P. (2021). Racism and health. https://www.apha.org/topics-and-issues/health-equity/racism-and-health

Kaiser Permanente Institute for Health Policy. (2016). *How racism makes people sick: A conversation with Camera Phyllis Jones, MD, MPH, PhD.*

Lewis, A. E. (2004). What group? Studying whites and whiteness in the era of color-blindness. *Sociological Theory, 22*(4), 623–646. https://doi.org/10.1111/j.0735-2751.2004.00237.x

McIntosh, P. (1989). White privilege: Unpacking the invisible knapsack. *Peace and Freedom*, July/August 18. https://psychology.umbc.edu/files/2016/10/White-Privilege_McIntosh-1989.pdf.

Nardi, D., Waite, R., Nowak, M., Hatcher, B., Hines-Martin, V., & Stacciarini, J.-M. (2020). Achieving health equity through eradicating structural racism in the United States: A call to action for nursing leadership. *Journal of Nursing Scholarship, 536*, 66–704.

National Action Committee International Perspectives: Women and Global Solidarity. http://www.aclrc.com/antiracism

Race Equity Tools. (2020). *Racial equity tools glossary.* https://www.racialequitytools.org/glossary

Schroeder, C., & DiAngelo, R. (2010). Addressing whiteness in nursing education. *Advances in Nursing Science, 33*(3), 244–255. https://doi.org/10.1097/ANS.0b013e3181eb41cf

Singleton, G. E. (2014). *Courageous conversations about race: A field guide for achieving equity in schools.* 2nd ed. Corwin.

Slater, K. (2021, February 4). What is systemic racism? *Today.* https://www.today.com/tmrw/what-systemic-racism-t207878

Trueman, S., Mills, J. E., & Usher, K. (2011). Racism in contemporary Australian nursing. *Aboriginal and Islander Health Worker Journal, 35*(5), 9–22.

Valderama-Wallace, C. P., & Apesoa-Varano, E. C. (2019). "Social justice is a dream": Tensions and contradictions in nursing education. *Public Health Nursing, 36*(5), 735–743.

Waite, R., & Nardi, D. (2017). Nursing colonialism in America: Implications for nursing leadership. *Journal of Professional Nursing, 35*, 18–25.

Waite, R., & Nardi, D. (2021). Understanding racism as a historical trauma that remains today: Implication for the nursing profession. *Creative Health Care Management, 27*(1), 19–24.

Whelan, J. C. (2015). *Does nursing have a diversity problem? Echoes & evidence nursing history and health policy blog.* University of Pennsylvania Barbara Bates Center for the Study of the History of Nursing. https://historian.nursing.upenn.edu/2015/02/26/diversity_nursing/

Williams-Washington, K. N. (2010). Historical trauma. In R. L. Hampton, T. P. Gullotta, & R. L. Crowel (Eds.), *Handbook of African American health* (pp. 31–50). The Guilford Press.

Williams-Washington, K. N., & Mills, C. P. (2018). African America historical trauma: Creating an inclusive measure. *Journal of Multicultural Counseling and Development. 46*(4), 246–263.

Zippia The Career Expert. (2021). *Chief nursing officer.* https://www.zippia.com/chief-nursing-officer-jobs/demographics/

2

The History of Race and Racism in the United States

"The plague of racism is insidious, entering into our minds as smoothly and quietly and invisibly as floating airborne microbes enter into our bodies to find lifelong purchase in our bloodstreams."
— Maya Angelou (1993)

Bestselling author Ta-Nehishi Coates writes, "Race is the child of racism, not the father" (Coates, 2015). Race and racism in the United States are inextricably intertwined and one cannot be discussed without the other. Race and racism are foundational to U.S. history and culture, yet many do not understand how deeply they are situated at our core. From our beginnings of conquest and slavery to the present day where racial designations signify the difference between life and death, the story of race and racism is a hard truth (Oluo, 2017). The hard truth must be told. The legacy of trauma from slavery and Jim Crow is essential to understanding present treatment and health of Black people in the United States. We will never be able to achieve a just and equitable society unless we understand how things came to be as they are.

After reading this chapter, the reader will be able to:

1. Discuss the social, political, and economic contexts of race
2. Explain the legacy of slavery in the United States and its impact on society today

3. Discuss the origin and persistence of popular and pervasive stereotypes of Black people
4. Explain how race and racism are used to justify oppression and inequality
5. Explain how structural racism maintains injustice and disadvantage
6. Discuss the ramifications of slavery and Jim Crow on current health disparities

WHAT IS RACE?

Race is a complex phenomenon. It has been studied and theorized for centuries with proposed conceptualizations that include biological, morphological, subspecies, geographic, population, kinship, and social underpinnings (Kendig, 2011; National Research Council, 2004).

Albeit nebulous and ill-defined, race produced dangerous pseudoscientific notions for categorizing humans that perpetuate prejudices, stereotypes, misconceptions, and false justifications for systemic injustices (Byrd & Clayton, 2001; Hoffman, 2004; Skibba, 2019).

In 2003, the Human Genome Project revealed that humans are 99.9% identical in their genetic makeup (National Institutes of Health, National Human Genome Research Institute, 2019). The concept of race is not born out of scientific discovery (Yudell et al., 2016). It is a human invention. **Race is a social construct** (Hoffman, 2004; Yudell et al., 2016). Moreover, race is a social, political, and legal construct rooted in a historical legacy of controlling resources by how one perceives, values, and behaves toward another group (Byrd & Clayton, 2001; Scott & Heslin, 2003).

Essential Facts

Racism
Assaults on the human spirit in the form of biases, prejudices, and an ideology of superiority that persistently causes moral suffering and perpetuate injustices and inequities (National Commission to Address Racism in Nursing, 2021)

RACISM FROM THE BEGINNING

The U.S. Constitution is the foundation of the American government and has been in existence since 1789 (U.S. Senate, n.d.). Article 1, Section II, Clause III of the Constitution, known as the Enumeration clause, apportioned representatives based on population density

(Legal Information Institute, n.d.). Every 10 years, each person living in the United States of America is counted to determine representation in Congress.

> *Representatives and direct Taxes shall be apportioned among the several States which may be included within this Union, according to their respective Numbers, which shall be determined by adding to the whole Number of free Persons, including those bound to Service for a Term of Years, and excluding Indians not taxed, three fifths of all other Persons.* (National Archives, 2019a)

The first census count contained only six questions (Eschner, 2017). It asked the name of the White male householder and the names of all other people in the household divided by categories: free White males 16 years of age and older, free White males under 16 years of age, free White females, all other free persons, and slaves (Eschner, 2017). Native Americans were not counted and only three out of every five slaves were counted (Eschner, 2017).

We can trace our current struggles with race and racism and the contemporary constructs of power, privilege, and white supremacy back to our nation's founding ideas of superiority versus inferiority, freedom versus oppression, representation versus exclusion, citizenship versus disenfranchisement, and advantage versus disadvantage (Harris, 1993). One had to be legally defined as White to be a citizen and had to own property to vote (Byrd & Clayton, 2001; Eschner, 2017; Harris, 1993).

Vocabulary

White supremacy: A political, economic, and cultural system in which Whites overwhelmingly control power and material resources, conscious and unconscious ideas of White superiority and entitlement are widespread, and relations of White dominance and non-White subordination are daily reenacted across a broad array of institutions and social settings (Ansley, 1989).

Antiblackness: The inability to recognize Black humanity and the disdain, disregard, and disgust for Black existence (Ross, 2020). It describes a specific kind of racism directed toward Black people that underscores the unique lived experience of Blacks in the United States (Ross, 2020). Antiblackness is the root of most oppression and racism in the United States (Jung & Vergas, 2021; Yes, 2020).

STRUCTURAL RACISM

Structural racism is not something that a few organizations or institutions choose to practice (Aspen Institute, 2016). Structural racism is the totality of ways in which societies foster racial discrimination through mutually reinforcing systems of housing, education, employment, earnings, benefits, credit, media, healthcare, and criminal justice (Bailey et al., 2017, p. 1453). These policies, patterns, and practices in turn reinforce discriminatory beliefs, values, and distribution of resources (Bailey et al., 2017, p 1453).

The legacies of slavery and Jim Crow are seen in structural racism (Owens & Fett, 2019). It is a feature of the social, economic, political, and healthcare systems in which we all function (Aspen Institute, 2016; Owens & Fett, 2019; Prather et al., 2018). Structural racism identifies dimensions of our history and culture that have allowed privileges associated with "whiteness" and disadvantages associated with "color" to endure and adapt over time (Aspen Institute, 2016).

The phrase "racism is baked into American society" and other similar metaphors convey the frustration and perplexity associated with the persistent, pervasive, and seemingly intractable inequities that exist in America today. The nursing profession must move beyond cultural humility to structural competency and shift the focus from individuals to institutions, systems, practices, and policies to address racism, bias, and discrimination as root causes of disparities and inequities in health, healthcare delivery, and healthcare outcomes (Davis & O'Brien, 2020). An understanding of structural racism must delineate and recount the experiences of Black people in North America. "The story of the African American is not only the quintessential American story but it's really the story that continues to shape who we are today" (Bunch, 2016).

AMERICAN SLAVERY

Slavery lasted for 246 years in the United States (Prather et al., 2018). Africans were brought to the Americas via the Middle Passage, stripped of human rights, and enslaved as chattel (Owens & Fett, 2019). Legalized chattel slavery was an inheritable status applied to enslaved women and their descendants (Owens & Fett, 2019). Treatment was brutal, degrading, and inhumane. Enslaved people were shipped, shackled, hanged, beaten, burned, mutilated, branded, and imprisoned (Byrd & Clayton, 2000; Chin, 2019). Rape and sexual abuse were common (Prather et al., 2018). Children born of sexual relations between any man and a Black woman were classified as slaves regardless of the father's race or status—a law known as partus sequitar ventrem (Owens & Fett, 2019). It was not uncommon for punishment to be inflicted just to reinforce dominance of the enslaver. Enslaved people had no defense or recourse (Chin, 2019; Higginbotham & Jacobs,

1992). Moreover, slave laws codified the status of enslaved people and the rights of enslavers. Enslaved people were deprived of an education and were not allowed to work for pay (Chin, 2019).

Enslaved Black people were exploited to build the world's most powerful economic system (Byrd & Clayton, 2000). Chattel slavery yielded more than $14 trillion and laid the groundwork for the concentration of wealth and power for Whites in America (Johnson, 2020). Whites built lineages of wealth for their families while enslaved Black people made money not for themselves but for the enslavers (Owens & Fett, 2019).

The pattern of inferior, inconsistent, and unfavorable healthcare for African American people in the United States can be traced back to the landing of Blacks as enslaved people in the Americas (Byrd & Clayton, 2000). Byrd and Clayton posit that health and healthcare delivery in the United States cannot be fully understood outside of the context of the nation's social, political, and economic environments.

Africans brought into North America for slavery during the slave trade in the 17th, 18th, and 19th centuries were in a deficient situation with regard to their health (Byrd & Clayton, 2000). The health professions must acknowledge their involvement in the institutions of slavery from its beginnings (Owens & Fett, 2019). This slave health deficit was due to the stresses and trauma of the slave trade (Byrd & Clayton, 2000; Hood, 2001). This included slave round ups and storage in slave castles on the African continent, deplorable conditions on ships during the Middle Passage across the Atlantic, and a harsh breaking-in period once in the Americas (Byrd & Clayton, 2000).

During the colonial period, laws clearly mandated the difference in treatment between White servants and Black enslaved people (Higginbotham, 1980). Detailed statutes outlined for the proper treatment of White servants did not exist for Black enslaved people (Higginbotham, 1980). The law was silent when it came to the care and treatment of Blacks (Higginbotham, 1980). Enslavers were allowed to feed, clothe, and treat enslaved Black people in whatever manner they saw fit (Higginbotham, 1980).

Hospitals were not favored by the colonist (Byrd & Clayton, 2001). The sick were cared for at home (Byrd & Clayton, 2001). Public almshouses provided a minimal level of care and quarantine for the worthy and unworthy poor (Byrd & Clayton, 2001). These poorhouses were overcrowded and racially segregated. The waiting lists for Blacks were extremely long. Thus, Black enslaved people took care of their own healthcare needs through a slave heath system composed of midwives, root doctors, and spiritual healers (Byrd & Clayton, 2001).

The question often posed is how did the early colonizers reconcile the Declaration of Independence, which states, "We hold these truths to be self-evident, that all men are created equal, that they are endowed by their Creator with certain unalienable Rights, that among these are Life, Liberty and the Pursuit of Happiness," with the brutality of chattel slavery (National Archives, 2019b)? After a long struggle of nearly 200 years after these basic human rights were proclaimed by the Declaration of Independence and guaranteed by the Constitution, the United States passed the initial civil rights legislation and formally recognized that Back and White people were equal under the law (Bowman, 2016).

This duality existed from the beginning. Notions that Africans were inferior, backward, and barbaric justified slavery (Olusoga, 2015). In fact, the origins of offensive contemporary stereotypes about Black people can be found in many of the justifications used for slavery (Bailey et al., 2021).

Essential Facts

The one drop rule is the centuries old practice, that persists today, of assigning minoritized status to mixed-race individuals (Blay, 2021; Bradt, 2010; Hickman, 1997). In 1920 the 14th Census adopted the one drop rule (Hickman, 1997); that is, a person of mixed blood is classified according to the non-White racial strain. Thus, a person of mixed White and Black heritage is classified as Black. Also known as the hypodescent rule, it dates back to a 1662 Virginia law on the treatment of mixed-race individuals and tells us about the hierarchical nature of race relations in the United States (Bradt, 2010). Children of a Black mother and White father were held bond or free only according to the condition of the mother (Hickman, 1997).

SCIENTIFIC RACISM

In addition to medicine, eugenics, and religion, scientific racism or pseudoscience was used to justify slavery (Ruane, 2019). The early colonist's belief of White superiority and Black inferiority was affirmed by an influx of pseudoscientific writings from the European medical and scientific community known as scientific racism (Scott & Heslin, 2003).

Prominent Harvard professors Samuel George Morton and Swiss-born Louis Agassiz sought to convince the medical and scientific community of the inferiority and subhuman status of the Black race (Menand, 2001/2002). The Slave Daguerreotypes of Louis Agassiz were designed to analyze the physical differences between European

Whites and African Blacks to prove the superiority of the White race (La, 2017).

Writings of Black biological, psychological, and intellectual inferiority proclaimed that Blacks were not expected to have normal medical outcomes (Scott & Heslin, 2003). As a result, Blacks suffered detrimental effects on health and healthcare in the 17th and 18th centuries and the legacy continues today (Prather et al., 2018; Scott & Heslin, 2003).

Race science creates categories of superior and inferior races based on the assumption that Blacks are inferior to Whites in the endowment of body and mind (Byrd & Clayton, 2001; Scott & Heslin, 2003). It espoused theories of physical and intellectual inferiority and likened Black people to animals, especially monkeys and apes (Byrd & Clayton, 2000). This thinking thrived in the 18th and 19th centuries and persists right up to present day (Bailey et al., 2021; Ruane, 2019). *Consider comedian "Roseanne Barr's use of an ape analogy in a tweet about Valerie Jarrett, an African American adviser to President Barack Obama, which led to the cancellation of Barr's ABC television show"* (Bailey et al., 2021; Ruane, 2019).

It is important to understand how medicine and science were implicit in the oppression, pathologizing, and dehumanization of Black bodies because it has huge reverberations and ramifications for the health and healthcare of Black people today (Opara et al., 2021). Racism, not race, is a risk factor for health disparities and poor health outcomes (Crear-Perry, 2018; Wallis, 2020). Josiah C. Nott was a South Carolina physician, anthropologist, and medical director in the Confederate army who, when speaking at a Southern Rights Association meeting in 1851, said "Their physical type is peculiar; their grade of intellect is greatly inferior; they are utterly wanting in moral and physical energy" (Ruane, 2019). This example features the pervasive and persistent stereotype of Blacks being lazy. It was believed that Blacks were less human and limited in their ability to feel pain (Hoffman et al., 2016). J. Marion Sims, known as the father of modern gynecology, repeatedly performed painful operations on enslaved Black women without anesthesia to perfect his vesicovaginal fistula repair (Bailey et al, 2021). Blacks continue to be systematically under-treated for pain due to false beliefs (Hoffman et al., 2016). Made-up diseases and false physiological peculiarities were ascribed to Blacks and taught by health professionals well into the 20th and 21st centuries (Bailey et al, 2021; Byrd & Clayton, 2001; Opara et al., 2021). In 1851 physician Samuel Cartwright described drapetomania, a disease that caused enslaved Africans to run away and was cured by whippings (Byrd & Clayton, 2001). Scientific racism contributed to the design of structural racism in healthcare and explicit and implicit bias among healthcare professionals that has prevailed for centuries (Reynolds, 2020).

Essential Facts

Jim Crow laws were passed immediately following the 13th Amendment which abolished slavery in the United States. Jim Crow laws are often referred to as slavery by another name as they restricted the freedom of Black people and imposed racial discrimination and segregation against Black people. They were named after Jim Crow, the fictional minstrel character who was created by a White actor Thomas Dartmouth Rice. Rice donned blackface and performed jokes and songs that mocked and made fun of enslaved Black people for the entertainment of White people (Ferris State University, n.d.; Lloyd Sealy Library, n.d.).

JIM CROW LAWS

In 1883, the Supreme Court ruled that the 1875 Civil Rights Act, which was created to allow equal access to public accommodations, was unconstitutional; this paved the way for Jim Crow laws. (Iowa.gov, n.d.). In 1896, the *Plessy v. Ferguson* Supreme Court decision upheld the constitutionality of racial segregation under the separate but equal doctrine (Iowa.gov, n.d.). The social determinants of health must be discussed within this context. Black codes marginalized Blacks and limited their freedom by denying them the right to vote, hold jobs, get an education, and other opportunities (PBS, 2021). Those who attempted to defy Jim Crow laws or Black codes were fined, arrested, jailed, and even suffered violence and death. Pig laws unfairly punished Blacks, who were poor and could not get jobs, for crimes such as stealing (PBS, 2021). Job opportunities were limited for Blacks yet vagrancy statutes made it a crime to be unemployed (PBS, 2021). Misdemeanors or minor offenses were treated as felonies with harsh sentences and fines (PBS, 2021). These codes still impact policing and prison in the 21st century (Alexander, 2020).

The Jim Crow era of legal discrimination and racial segregation during the late 1800s and into the early 20th century created another damaging legacy for the health and healthcare of Blacks (Scott & Heslin, 2003). The U.S. healthcare system evolved in the 100-year period of Jim Crow laws that enforced racial segregation in public services and facilities (Largent, 2018; Scott & Heslin, 2003). During this period, Blacks were required to use separate and substandard healthcare facilities (Scott & Heslin, 2003). Denying the continued impact of historically institutionalized racism in the provision of care in the health professions only risks further perpetuating it in our current system (Largent, 2018; Scott & Henslin, 2003). Therefore the hard truth must be recounted.

Jim Crow laws and the colonial backlash from the Bacon Rebellion in 1676 are said to be two events in history designed to ensure divisions between Blacks and Whites and provide the basis for American concepts of race, racism, and white supremacy (Tatum, 2017).

Harsh, cruel, unbelievable, ugly, and shameful, this chapter of history gives the necessary hard truth. We are all at varying stages in terms of our knowledge, understanding, and willingness to connect the past to the present. The first step in dismantling systemic racism is knowing the true history of America. Once you know the history you are better positioned to take steps toward creating a more just and equitable society by mitigating your implicit biases and minimizing your microaggressions. History is something that all Americans must own. You can see from reading this chapter how the dominate prevailing culture has influenced our thoughts, beliefs, practices, and policies. It is more apparent now that there is a standoff between our recent attention to promoting heath equity and social justice and the old, ingrained policies, practices, and social mores of bias and discrimination.

Critical Thinking Questions

Connecting the Past to the Present

1. Reflect on your comfort level when reading about slavery in America. What made you feel the way you were feeling?
2. What are the consequences of slavery and the Jim Crow era on the health and wealth of Blacks in America today?
3. Does reading this chapter give you a better understanding of the terms white supremacy and antiblackness?
4. Why is it necessary to assign the case of Simkins v. Moses H. Cone Memorial Hospital as required reading for assignments related to the Hill-Burton Act of 1946 and development of the U.S. healthcare system?

CASE STUDY

I walked into my assigned patient's room and said, "Good morning, Mrs. Walker." Before I could say anything else, Mrs. Walker looked at me and said, "My breakfast tray is over there on the table." I responded, "Mrs. Walker, I am not here for your breakfast tray, I am your student nurse for today." The patient responded, "Come over here and let me see your badge."

Despite being dressed in the required student nurse uniform, that prominently displayed my academic affiliation, my patient thought I was from dietary services, there to collect her tray. After learning that I was her student nurse, she then needed to see my credentials.

This was my first encounter with racism and patient bias. I was being judged and questioned because of the color of my skin. I was saddened, hurt, angry, and disappointed.

I am excited every day that I walk into the hospital to take care of patients because I get to live my dream, fulfill my purpose, and use my knowledge and skills to make a difference in the lives of others. I have an obligation as a nurse to treat everyone with dignity and respect and to give them the best care possible.

Although my enthusiasm had not waned and my commitment to provide the best care possible to all patients remained intact after the encounter with Mrs. Walker, I could not shake my feelings of hurt, anger, and disappointment. I had been wounded. I was crushed. I wanted to tell my clinical instructor about the incident. However, we had never discussed issues of race and racism in class. I did not know if she would understand. I wanted to discuss it in post-conference however, I was not sure how it would be received as I was the only student of color in that clinical rotation.

I wondered how often the nurses on that floor encountered discriminatory behaviors from patients. I felt as if I were not standing up for other nurses of color by not saying something to the nursing leadership on that unit.

By being my best and providing the best care possible for that patient, maybe, just maybe, I showed her that I am qualified and capable. However, why should I have to prove myself because of the color of my skin? In addition to feeling sad, hurt, angry, and disappointed, I felt guilty and confused.

Case Study Questions

1. As an educator or nurse manager have you ever witnessed a nurse or nursing student subjected to patient racism, bias, or discrimination? If so, how did you handle the situation?
2. In the future if you witness a nurse or nursing student being subjected to patient racism, bias, or discrimination how will you handle it?

3. Have you ever addressed or reported patient racism, bias, or discrimination? How did your organization handle the situation?
4. If you were the clinical instructor or nurse manager, how would you approach the student after the incident with Mrs. Walker?

REFERENCES

Alexander, M. (2020). *The new Jim Crow: Mass incarceration in the age of colorblindness*. New York: New Press.

Angelou, M. (1993). *Wouldn't take nothing for my journey now*. Random House.

Ansley, F. L. (1989). Stirring the ashes: Race class and the future of civil rights scholarship. *Cornell Law Review, 74*(6), 993–1077. https://scholarship.law.cornell.edu/cgi/viewcontent.cgi?article=3431&context=clr

Aspen Institute. (2016, July 11). 11 terms you should know to better understand structural racism. https://www.aspeninstitute.org/blog-posts/structural-racism-definition/

Bailey, Z. D., Krieger, N., Agénor, M., Graves, J., Linos, N., & Bassett, M. T. (2017). Structural racism and health inequities in the USA: Evidence and interventions. *Lancet, 389*(10077), 1453–63.

Bailey, Z. D., Feldman, J. M., & Bassett, M. T. (2021). How structural racism works – Racist policies as a root cause of U.S. *Racial Health Inequities. New England Journal of Medicine, 384*(8), 768–773. https://doi.org/10.1056/nejmms2025396

Blay, Y. (2021). *One drop shifting the lens on race*. Beacon Press.

Bowman, L. G. (2016, July 1). *The paradox of the Declaration of Independence*. Aspen Institute. https://www.aspeninstitute.org/blog-posts/every-american-know-paradox-declaration-independence/

Bradt, S. (2010). *Science and technology. One-drop rule persists*. The Harvard Gazette. https://news.harvard.edu/gazette/story/2010/12/one-drop-rule-persists/

Bunch, L. G. III. (2016, September). The definitive story of how the national museum of African American history and culture came to be. https://www.smithsonianmag.com/smithsonian-institution/definitive-story-national-museum-african-american-history-culture-came-be-180960125/

Byrd, M. W., & Clayton, L. A. (2001). Race, medicine, and health care in the United States: A historical survey. *Journal f the National Medical Association*, 3(3 Suppl), 11S–34S. https://www.ncbi.nlm.nih.gov/pmc/articles/PMC2593958/

Byrd, M. W., & Clayton, L. A. (2000). *An American health dilemma: A medical history of African Americans and the problem of race; beginnings to 1900* (Vol. 1). Routledge.

Chin, W. (2019). Legal inequality: Law, the legal system, and the lessons of the Black experience in America. *Hastings Race and Poverty Law Review, 16*, 109–140.

Coates, T. (2015). *Between the world and me*. Spiegel & Grau.

Crear-Perry, J. (2018, April 11). Race isn't a risk factor in maternal health. Racism is. Rewire News Group. https://rewirenewsgroup.com/article/2018/04/11/maternalhealth-replace-race-with-racism/

Davis, S., & O'Brien, A.-M. (2020). Let's talk about racism. Building structural competency in nursing. *Academic Medicine, 5*, S58–S65. https://doi.org/10.1097/ACM.0000000000003688

Eschner, K. (2017, August, 2). The first us census only asked six questions. https://www.smithsonianmag.com/smart-news/first-us-census-only-asked-six-questions-180964234/

Ferris State University. (n.d.). What was Jim Crow. Jim Crow Museum of Racist Memorabilia. https://www.ferris.edu/jimcrow/what.htm

Harris, C. L. (1993). Whiteness as property. *Harvard Law Review, 106*(8), 1707–1791. https://www.jstor.org/stable/1341787?seq=1#metadata_info_tab_contents

Hickman, C. B. (1997). The devil and the one drop rule: Racial categories. *African Americans, and the U.S. Census. 5*(5), 1161–1265. https://repository.law.umich.edu/cgi/viewcontent.cgi?article=4313&context=mlr

Higginbotham, A. L. (1980). *In the matter of color, race and the American legal process: The colonial period*. New York: Oxford University Press.

Higginbotham, A. L., & Jacobs, A. E. (1992). The law only as a enemy: The legitimization of racial powerless through the colonial and antebellum criminal laws of Virginia. *North Carolina Law Review, 70*(4), 969–1070.

Hoffman, S. (2004). Is there a place for race as a legal concept. *Faculty Publications, 227*, 1093–1159. https://scholarlycommons.law.case.edu/faculty_publications/227

Hoffman, K. M., Trawalter, S., Axt, J. R., & Oliver, M. N. (2016). Racial bias in pain assessment and treatment recommendations, and false beliefs about biological differences between Blacks and Whites. *Proceedings of the National Academies Science of the United States, 113*(16), 4296–4301.

Hood, R. G. (2001). The "slave health deficit:" The case for reparations to bring health parity to African Americans. *The Journal of the National Medical Association, 3*(1), 1–5.

Iowa.gov. (n.d.). Iowa Department of Human Rights. Jim Crow Laws. https://humanrights.iowa.gov/cas/saa/african-american-culture-history/jim-crow-laws

Johnson, R. L. (2020, June 1). *Robert L. Johnson, founder of black entertainment television and the RLJ companies, issues statement and full proposal for full Black American reparations*. The RLJ Companies. https://www.prnewswire.com/news-releases/robert-l-johnson-founder-of-black-entertainment-television-and-the-rlj-companies-issues-statement-and-proposal-for-full-black-american-reparations-301068343.html

Jones, C. P. (2021). *Racism and health*. American Public Health Association. https://www.apha.org/topics-and-issues/health-equity/racism-and-health

Jung, M. K. & Vergas, J. C. H. (eds). (2021). Antiblackness. Duke University Press.

Kendig, C. (2011). Race as a physiosocial phenomenon. *History Philosophy Life Science, 33*, 191–222. https://www.jstor.org/stable/23335116

La, S. (2017, July 3). Black lives, White lies: The Black photographer has always been disregarded by the new world. The Race Card. *Afropunk*. https://afropunk.com/2017/07/black-lives-white-lens-black-photographer-always-disregarded-new-world/

Largent, E.A. (2018). Public health, racism, and the lasting impact of hospital segregation. *Public Health Reports, 133*(6), 715–720.

Legal Information Institute (n.d.). Cornell Law School. https://www.law.cornell.edu/constitution/articlei

Lloyd Sealy Library. (n.d.). American history: The civil war and reconstruction: Amendments, acts and codes of reconstruction. https://guides.lib.jjay.cuny.edu/c.php?g=288398&p=1922458

Menand, L. (2001/2002). Morton, Agassiz, and the origins of scientific racism in the United States. *Journal of Blacks in Higher Education, 34*, 110–113. http://www.jstor.org/stable/3134139

National Archives. (2019a, November, 19). America's founding documents. The constitution of the United States: A transcription. https://www.archives.gov/founding-docs/constitution-transcript

National Archives. (2019b, November, 19). America's founding documents. Declaration of Independence: A Transcription. https://www.archives.gov/founding-docs/declaration-transcript

National Commission to Address Racism in Nursing. (2021). Defining racism. https://www.nursingworld.org/~49f737/globalassets/practiceandpolicy/workforce/commission-to-address-racism/final-defining-racism-june-2021.pdf

National Institutes of Health, National Human Genome Research Institute. (2019, October 7). The human genome project. https://www.genome.gov/human-genome-project

National Research Council. (2004). Measuring racial discrimination. *The National Academies Press*. https://doi.org/10.17226/10887

Oluo, I. (2017, September 5). *There is no middle ground between racism and justice*. The Establishment. https://theestablishment.co/there-is-no-middle-ground-between-racism-and-justice-8838f14e46a3/index.html

Olusoga, D. (2015, September 8). The roots of European racism lie in the slave trade, colonialism – And Edward Long. *The Guardian*.

Opara, I. N., Riddles-Jones, L., & Allen, N. (2021). Modern day drapetomania: Calling out scientific racism. *Journal of General Internal Medicine, 37*(1), 225–226.

Owens, D. C., & Fett, S. M. (2019). Black maternal and infant health: Historical legacies of slavery. *American Journal of Public Health, 109*(10), 1342–1345. https://doi.org/10.2105/AJPH.2019.305243

PBS. (2021). Slavery by another name. Black codes and pig laws. https://www.pbs.org/tpt/slavery-by-another-name/themes/black-codes/

Prather, C., Fuller, T. R., Jeffries, W.L., Marchall, K.J., Howell, A.V., Belyue-Umole, A., & King, W. (2018). Racism, African American Women and their sexual and reproductive health: A review of historical and contemporary evidence and implications for health equity. *Health Equity, 2*(1), 249–259. http://online.liebertpub.com/doi/10.1089/heq.2017.0045

Reynolds, P. P. (2020, January 9). UVA and the history of race: Eugenics, the racial integrity act, health disparities. *UVA Today*. https://news.virginia.edu/content/uva-and-history-race-eugenics-racial-integrity-act-health-disparities

Ross, K. M. (2020). Call it what it is: Anti-Blackness. https://www.nytimes.com/2020/06/04/opinion/george-floyd-anti-blackness.html

Ruane, M. E. (2019, April 30). A brief history of the enduring phony science that perpetuates white supremacy. *The Washington Post*. https://www.washingtonpost.com/local/a-brief-history-of-the-enduring-phony-science-that-perpetuates-white-supremacy/2019/04/29/20e6aef0-5aeb-11e9-a00e-050dc7b82693_story.html

Scott, R. P., & Heslin, K. C. (2003). Historical perspectives in the care of African Americans with cardiovascular disease. *The Annals of Thoracic Surgery, 76*(4), S1348–1355.

Skibba, R. (2019, May, 20). The disturbing resilience of scientific racism. *Smithsonian Magazine*. https://www.smithsonianmag.com/science-nature/disturbing-resilience-scientific-racism-180972243/

Tatum, D. C. (2017). Donald Trump and the legacy of Beacon's Rebellion. *Journal of Black Studies, 48*(7), 651–674. https://www.jstor.org/stable/10.2307/26574529

United States Senate (n.d.). https://www.senate.gov/artandhistory/history/common/generic/ConstitutionDay.htm

Willis, C. (2020, June 12). Why racism, not race, is a risk factor for dying of COVID-19. Scientific American. https://www.scientificamerican.com/article/why-racism-not-race-is-a-risk-factor-for-dyingof-covid-191/

Yes. (2020). Let's talk about anti-Blackness. https://www.yesmagazine.org/education/2020/04/07/lets-talk-about-anti-blackness

Yudell, M., Roberts, D., DeSalle, R., & Tishkoff, S. (2016). Taking race out of human genetics. *Science, 351*(6273), 564–565. https://science.sciencemag.org/content/351/6273/564

3

Racism: Root Cause of Social and Structural Determinants of Health

"Racism is one of the most divisive forces in our society. Racial legacies of the past continue to haunt current policies and practices that create unfair disparities between minority and majority groups."

—Advisory Board to the President's Initiative on Race, 1998

It has been over two decades since the President's Advisory Board (Franklin & The Advisory Board to the President's Initiative on Race, 1998) called out racism and bias as root causes of inequality. Despite decades of federal planning and myriad institutional efforts to reduce disparities, we still not made any significant progress. In an interview with O'Hara (2018), Dr. David Williams, Professor at Harvard, suggested that the problem persists because of our society's "empathy gap.": "'For most Americans, we do not care' what happens to black people" (p. 5). As we explore the complicated reasons for the persistent racial and ethnic disparities in America, let us reflect on Dr. Williams's words and think about how knowledge and attitudes play a role in the action and/or inaction to achieve health equity.

After reading this chapter, the reader will be able to:

1. Learn and apply key terms related to racial health and wealth disparities
2. Understand how individual, institutional, and structural racism contribute to health disparities and unequal life chances

3. Learn strategies for addressing the root causes of health disparities and promoting health equity

The first step for clinicians is to become familiar with key terms related to health and wealth disparities (Table 3.1).

INDIVIDUAL-LEVEL BIAS AND RACISM AS SOCIAL DETERMINANTS OF HEALTH

As early as 2009, Jones et al. identified racism as a social determinant of equity and a key factor in optimizing the health and well-being of clients, families, and communities of color. More recently, Matthew (2018) cited a large of body of research that has demonstrated the impact of physician-implicit and -explicit bias on client/provider communication, provider decision-making, and racial disparities in health outcomes.

Hakima Payne, MSN, RN, and former L&D nurse, provided insight as well on how bias impacts clinician attitudes toward non-White clients, "The conversations that took place behind the nurse's station that just made assumptions; a lot of victim-blaming—'If those people would only do blah, blah, blah, things would be different'" (Martin & Montagne, 2017, p. 4).

Over two decades ago, Tervalon and Murray-Garcia (1998) recognized the dangers of implicit bias and proposed that health professionals shift away from the focus on *cultural competence* and toward the development of *cultural humility*. Practicing under this approach, clinicians would recognize that:

1. We all have inherent bias and be aware of them during our client/clinician interactions.
2. We are in a position of power as the healthcare professional and need to consciously work to create equality in those interactions.
3. We need to partner with community groups that work to promote health equity.

Practicing cultural humility, however, requires each of us to not only recognize our biases, but also to recognize the power and privilege we hold as healthcare professionals. Unlike the prior approach of cultural competence, culturally humility emphasizes that there is *no competency/end point* to be gained, but rather "a lifelong commitment to self-evaluation and critique, to redressing power imbalances" (Tervalon & Murray-Garcia, 1998, p. 123).

Table 3.1

Key Terms Related to Social and Structural Determinants of Health

Term	Definition	Example
Black, Indigenous, and People of Color (BIPOC)	Global term for persons of color in the United States	Minoritized groups that have come together in solidarity to undo White supremacy and ensure racial justice such as "The BIPOC Project (n.d.)"
Health disparities	Differences in incidence or prevalence of health conditions across different groups. Stratified groups can include one or more of the following: race, gender, religious affiliation, sexual orientation, socioeconomic status, neighborhoods	Native American women are twice as likely and Black women are three times as likely as White women to die from pregnancy-related complications (Petersen et al., 2019)
Health equity	In contrast to equality, equity is about identifying and providing each person with the necessary supports to live to their full potential	*Wrap-around services* in our public schools to address the cognitive, psychological, and socioemotional needs of children and to help families connect with local support services (Love et al., 2019)
Minority-serving institutions (MSI)	Institutions that have a mission to primarily support minority students. Examples include Hispanic-serving institutions (HSI), historically Black colleges and universities (HBCU), Tribal colleges and universities (TCU), Asian American and Pacific Islander-serving nstitutions (AAPISI)	Famous HBCUs: Spelman, Howard, Morehouse. A recent study by Gallup-US Funds found that Black graduates from HBCUs were more likely than those from a non-HBCU to be thriving economically and to report feeling excited, supported, and mentored at their university (Seymour & Ray, 2015)
Predominately White Institutions (PWI)	Institutions where the majority of the leadership and employees are White (Brown & Dancy, 2010) and whose histories, policies and practices center around the White majority (Holmes et al., 2000)	Being at a PWI college or university where minority students risk feeling marginalized by the dominate culture (Bourke, 2016, p. 14) and feeling isolated or excluded (Griffith et al., 2019)

(continued)

Table 3.1

Key Terms Related to Social and Structural Determinants of Health (*continued*)

Term	Definition	Example
Purpose built Communities (PBC)	A network that started in 2009 and includes over 25 communities that have leveraged local leaders, community members, and other committed stakeholders to improve racial and economic equity (PBC, 2021).	The East Lake community near Atlanta that was transformed from a "war zone to a national model" through the collaborative efforts of philanthropists and local citizen groups (PBC, 2012).
School-to-prison pipeline	How disciplinary policies and practices disproportionately target Black youth and lead to higher rates of juvenile incarceration and lower graduation rates (Nelson & Lind, 2015)	The presence of police/school resource officers in schools has increased over the last two decades and federal data indicate that while Black youth were 16% of the children enrolled in the 2011–2012 school year, they comprised 31% of in-school arrests (Nelson & Lind, 2015)
Social determinants of health	Factors in our daily lives that can directly and/or indirectly impact one's health and well-being such as housing, food, and neighborhood	Children born in the Maryland and Virginia suburbs of Washington, DC, will live on average 6 to 7 years more than those born in the city (Robert Wood Johnson Foundation, 2013)
Structural determinants of equity or inequity	Those elements involved in societal decision-making (e.g., structures, policies, practices, values, and norms) (Jones, 2018)	The 1994 Violent Crime Control and Law Enforcement Act, which led to disproportionate rates of incarceration in the Black community (Lussenhop, 2016)
Toxic stress	The negative stress response from adverse childhood experiences: The stress can lead to lifelong changes in the developing brain and other body organs (Shonkoff et al., 2012)	Adults with a score of four or more on the ACEs Quiz (Center on the Developing Child, n.d.) are significantly more likely to suffer from heart disease, alcoholism and/or to attempt suicide (Felitti et al. 1998). An updated screening tool with additional questions can be found at The Philadelphia ACE Project (2021) (www.philadelphiaaces.org)

(continued)

Table 3.1

Key Terms Related to Social and Structural Determinants of Health (*continued*)

Term	Definition	Example
Weathering	A term to explain the cumulative cellular damage that results from the stress effect of racist experiences on Black women's health (Geronimus et al., 2010)	Even after controlling for income and education, Black women experience significant disparities in maternal morbidity and mortality: "When the Bough Breaks" (California Newsreel, 2008a)

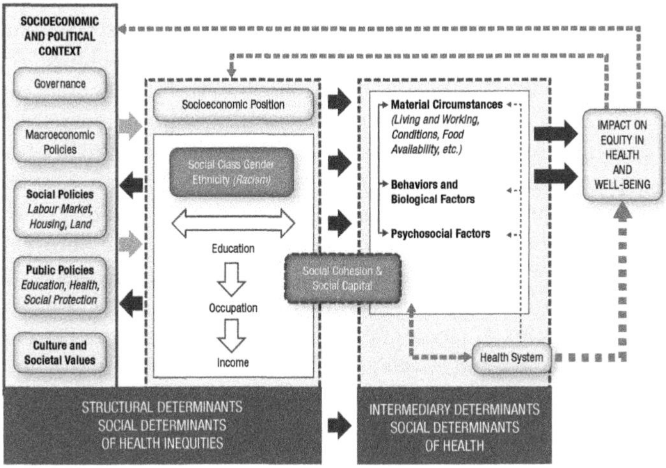

Figure 3.1 Commission on Social Determinants of Health Conceptual Framework.
Source: Reproduced with permission from Solar, O., & Irwin, A. (2010). *A conceptual framework for action on the social determinants of health: Social Determinants of Health Discussion Paper 2 (Policy and Practice)*. World Health Organization.

STRUCTURAL AND SOCIAL DETERMINANTS OF HEALTH

In 2010, the World Health Organization (WHO), among others, further shifted our collective gaze from the impact of the provider/client encounter to the critical role that structural and social determinants have on health and health inequities. Figure 3.1 presents the WHO's framework highlighting the significant impact that governmental policy, society's cultures and values, and one's social and economic position have on an individual's health and well-being (Solar & Irwin, 2010). What is striking and important to note is the interplay around the power to make change: a process that requires both a community's own agency (i.e., social cohesion and capital) and the acknowledged responsibility on the part of the government/state (i.e., socioeconomic and political context) (Solar & Irwin, 2010; Figure 3.1).

Soon after the WHO developed its framework, physician scientists Metzl and Hansen (2014) recognized the need for medical education to adopt a new curriculum based on a "structural competency framework" in order to further acknowledge and address the root causes of health and wealth inequalities. Drawing from a diverse set of disciplines and theories (e.g., sociology, critical race theory, economics, urban planning) this paradigm-shifting approach requires clinicians to not only recognize "the social and economic structures that contribute to inequities," but to also "mobilize" for equity and social change (Metzl et al., 2018, p. 190). Hansen and Metzl (2017) recently found that using a structural competency framework to teach health professions students has led to innovative partnerships-not only across disciplines, but also across the various sectors involved in health justice. Metzl et al. (2018) have now called for clinicians and health systems to test the impact of this framework on clinical practice and client health outcomes.

Following are some tools that can help clinicians and health professions students to incorporate these structural competencies into practice. O'Gurek and Henke (2018) provide an excellent overview of several of them:

- The PRAPARE Screening Tool (2022) which screens clients on 17 core social determinants of health (SDH) measures and another four optional measures and can be used as part of an organization/community's overall plan to "prepare," "assess," and/or "respond" to SDH data (https://prapare.org/the-prapare-screening-tool/)
- The American Association of Family Physician's (2022) "The EveryONE project toolkit" which includes:
  - An 11-item "Social Needs Screening Tool"
  - A "Neighborhood Navigator Tool" to help identify community resources in your area
  - A fillable-PDF to create your "Patient Social Needs Action Plan"
- The Centers for Medicare & Medicaid Services (2020) Accountable Health Communities Health-Related Social Needs Screening Tool, which includes a 10-item tool and supplemental questions

Another important tool is the Structural Vulnerability Assessment Tool (Bourgois et al., 2017), which assesses for vulnerabilities related to:

- Financial, housing, environmental, food access, and/or legal issues
- Social isolation and/or interpersonal danger
- Education and literacy
- Discrimination (race, gender, and/or sexual identity, other).

Of note, the tool also has a section for the clinician to engage in a moment of self-reflection to ask how their biases and/or those of their colleagues might lead to the client not receiving equitable care and/or increase feelings of distrust on the part of the client.

Essential Facts

"83,000 excess deaths each year. That's the equivalent of a major airliner filled with Black passengers falling out of the sky every single day, every year." (California Newsreel, 2008b, p. 10)

STRUCTURAL RACISM

Not since the Civil Rights Movement, has there been such a societal groundswell calling for racial justice and a critical examination of structural barriers that have greatly limited the life chances of most Black Americans (Table 3.2). As cited by Jones (2018), the United Nations Committee on the Elimination of Racial Discrimination (UNCERD) identified several structural barriers to achieving health and wealth equity in the United States including:

- Racial profiling
- Residential segregation
- Educational achievement gap
- Disproportionate incarceration
- Unequal access to healthcare

Jones (2018) further noted that in order to effectively address health equity we need to:

- First, name it, for when we don't, we become complicit in societal denial.
- Next, assess how is it operating here (e.g., community, state, national levels).
- Finally, organize and strategize with partnering institutions.

Table 3.2

Structural Racism Has Contributed to Disparities Via:

Term	Definition	Example
Environmental racism	Zoning and placement of toxic industrial plants in historically Black neighborhoods (Garza, 2021)	Dallas case with Mountain of Shingles describes the lasting effects of red-lining in a Dallas community and the lack of attention by city leaders to address the illegal dumping of toxic shingles in an historically Black neighborhood (Fears, 2020)
Food deserts	Usually located in urban areas where hypersegregated Black neighborhoods lack access to affordable/ high-quality grocery stores	Even when neighborhoods were matched by socioeconomic status, Black neighborhoods have higher access to fast food and less access to fresh fruits and vegetables than White neighborhoods (Landrine & Corral, 2009)
Healthcare deserts	Geographic areas where there is a lack of access to care (e.g., rural areas or underresourced urban areas)	Tung et al. (2019) found that Black majority census tracts were the only race/ethnic group areas to consistently have "trauma care deserts"

Essential Facts

"Where we live, learn, work and play has a greater impact on how long and how well we live than access to physicians [/clinicians]." – Dr. David R. Williams (cited by Anderson, 2012, p. 21)

STRATEGIES FOR ADDRESSING RACISM

Individual Level Action

In the wake of America's need to fully recognize the problem of structural *racism* in healthcare, Legha et al. (2020) developed "Five Core Components" for developing an "Antiracist Approach" to clinical care, which include:

- "Learning the legacy of racism" in healthcare so we recognize it and don't unintentionally "perpetuate it"
- Acknowledging the "racist" bias that exists within ourselves and our institutions in order to become an "antiracist"

- Slowing down our actions so we have time to assess our implicit bias reactions and how they might be impacting our clinical engagement and decision-making processes
- Identifying and opposing racism at the individual, institutional, and policy levels
- Encouraging our health systems to become anchor institutions that work to increase human capital and economic equity

Additional Strategies Might Include

- Learn more about implicit bias through the free series created by the Michigan Health Council (2020)
- Begin each clinical encounter with intentionality: Use your assessment skills to mindfully draw your attention to communication patterns with clients and colleagues. The Institute for Healthcare Improvement (IHI, 2017) offers an excellent tool called "Liberation in the Exam Room" to help clinicians and teams work together to create equitable and safe care settings
- Offer to partner with a colleague to peer evaluate each other's communication patterns. Think about it as "having each other's back" by sharing your observations with compassionate candor. Of importance is having a trusted colleague who is willing to engage in such a difficult, but critical opportunity for improving one's practice
- Note any patterns in team meetings about how cases are presented. Consider removing "race" from the SB in SBAR (Situation, Background, Assessment, Recommendation). For example, consider why we think the "race" of a client is an important component of the contextual information?

Institutional-Level Action

Brady (2014) provides an excellent case study for the trauma that results when institutions lack specific policies and practices to address situations where a racist patient refuses care from a BIPOC healthcare professional. Nurses can reduce healthcare harm by advocating for our practice sites to develop policies and practices that make explicit that we do not tolerate racial discrimination. As part of the training process, employees should have seminar time to reflect on the organization's values for providing racially equitable care, and how they plan to uphold these values.

Anstey and Wright (2014) also provide an excellent exemplar with their "Caregiver Preference Guideline" to illustrate how the Ontario health system responds to a client request for a provider based on a specific *social attribute*. In brief, steps in their process include:

- Provider assesses client's reasons for the specific request
- Provider discusses request with manager/supervisor
- Manager meets with client (caregiver has choice to attend), further assesses the situation, and then counsels the client on the institution's commitment to equity and antidiscrimination

Wyatt et al. (2016) similarly developed a white paper on behalf of IHI to assist institutions with their efforts to achieve health equity. The guide offers a five-component framework, a self-assessment tool to measure their efforts, as well as an exemplar on how one healthcare organization implemented its health equity initiative.

Finally, The Ohio State Wexner Medical Center (2020) provides institutions with a roadmap of their Antiracism Action Plan that involves the five steps of "elevate," "engage," "equip," "empower," and "evaluate" as part of an institution's efforts to eradicate structural racism and promote health equity. The program invites all stakeholders/providers, employees, students, patients, and community members to become part of the solution. The program includes not only tools and resources, but also opportunities for people to engage together in dialogue and work toward action.

Additional Strategies for Promoting Health Equity

- Suggest creating a task force to assess for disparities in client health outcomes. Employees across the practice setting should be invited to be a part of the process of reviewing the data, identifying root causes, and in developing plans for action.
- Nurses can also collaborate with existing organizational committees such as a quality improvement committee or a nursing research/evidence-based practice council. A Plan-Do-Check-Act (PDCA) model can guide the process. Questions to guide the interdisciplinary teams might include assessing for racial disparities in:
  - Patient morbidity and mortality
  - Which clients are referred for preventive/screening tests
  - Patient understanding of their healthcare/discharge instructions
  - Client ability to self-manage their chronic health conditions
  - How clients access healthcare: emergency, urgent, versus primary care
- Clinical nurse educators and nurse leaders can also reach out to the National League for Nursing/Walden University College of Nursing Institute for Social Determinants of Health and Social Change, which is an innovative partnership designed to help

educators and organizational leaders build their institutional capacity to promote health equity and structural change (Davis, 2022). In particular, the Institute's Leadership Academy was created to develop leaders and cultivate leadership competencies to (a) competently and confidently integrate SDH and social change into programs and curricula, and (b) engage in research and other scholarly activities with broad dissemination (Davis, 2022).

- Nurses can also encourage their institutions to utilize the National Center on Domestic Violence, Trauma and Mental Health's "Tools for Transformation" toolkit to create a more "accessible, culturally responsive, trauma-informed" healthcare organization (Warshaw et al., 2018).
  - Of particular importance to providers is an understanding that our nation's "historical trauma, structural oppression, and identity-based violence" can directly impact our organization's own culture and processes (Warsaw et al., 2018, p. 7).
  - As part of an antiracism practice, nurses can ask their organizations to create an interdisciplinary work group to review the toolkit and then propose a process for implementing changes system wide.

On a final note, let us reflect on the changes that have occurred in healthcare after the landmark report, "To Err is Human" (Institute of Medicine [IOM] Committee on Quality of Health Care in America et al., 2000), and in particular the concepts of "culture of safety" and "just culture." From the IOM report, organizations and health professions learned that promoting quality and safety required systems to move beyond blaming the individual and toward recognizing that being human means providers are fallible and thus inherently at risk for making mistakes. In a similar context, we need to recognize that we live and work in a society that has not yet fully recognized its 400 years of racism, bias, and discrimination (David, 2014). As a result, both explicit and implicit bias are credible threats to the health and well-being of our colleagues and clients of color. So how can we create a "just culture" for addressing racism in our practice setting? Some suggestions:

- Does your institution have a person/committee to whom you can report incidents of bias or discrimination? And if so, are they set up for promoting positive change versus individual punishment, blame, and shame?
- Is there a policy in place for when a racist patient doesn't want a provider of color? If not, consider a model as outlined by Anstey and Wright (2014) and create a similar algorithm for how to safely address these requests.

- Remember to include key BIPOC stakeholders (e.g., providers, administrators, community members of color) when developing your institution's policies and processes.
- Nurses can become part of the solution by ensuring that our colleagues' and institutions' patterns and practices do not violate Section 1557 of the 2010 Patient Protection and Affordable Care Act, which has further strengthened federal enforcement against discrimination in healthcare (Matthew, 2018).

Essential Facts

Many Black Americans are tired—tired of seeing the injustices continue and while they might be glad to have White allies, they still wonder, "Where have you been?" (Falson, 2020).

Addressing Structural Racism

As more and more clinicians and public health professionals call attention to structural racism as a public health crisis (American Public Health Association [APHA], 2020; Moore, 2020), we nurses must recognize our own ethical obligation to address it. Nurses can seek out examples from other healthcare and professional organizations to guide our efforts and/or seek to partner with fellow nurses in our own specialty organization. For example, school nurses could use the National Association of School Nurses' (NASN, 2020) Position Brief, *Eliminate Racism to Optimize Student Health and Learning*, as a guide for collaborating with their school colleagues and creating an antiracism school culture. Strategies suggested by the NASN (2020) include:

- Examining the disparities in academic achievement and disciplinary cases
- Asking and empathetically listening to those who have experienced discrimination/racism
- Identifying evidence-based curricular interventions to improve diversity, equity, and inclusion in the school
- Collaborating with colleagues and teachers to increase student feelings of connectedness and belonging

We can also partner with public health departments, federally qualified health centers (FQHC) and other service agencies to address SDHs that are most pressing to our communities. Table 3.3 provides examples of successful action.

Table 3.3

Examples of Successful Action

Initiative	Description	Action
Greensboro Health Disparities Collaborative	Partnership with Greensboro and UNC Chapel Hill to address racial disparities among patients diagnosed with cancer	Accountability for Cancer Care Through Undoing Racism and Equity (ACCURE) Project: Staff offered training in health disparities and specialty nurse navigators followed clients from diagnosis to end of treatment. Black/White disparities disappeared in the intervention group, but remained the same in the control groups (Hostetter & Klein, 2018)
Ward 8 Community Economic Development Plan (W8CED)	Collective group of DC stakeholders committed to building sustainable economic empowerment. The group shifts the paradigm from a "deficit-based mindset to an asset-based stance" (www.ward8cedplan.com, n.d.)	The organization has partnered with Streetwyze.com, community residents and several health and social service agencies to map community businesses and services
Fairfax County's "Live Health Fairfax" Initiative (2018)	Created a five-year plan to guide cross-sector partnership with community member engagement to promote health equity	Established a community health dashboard for residents and partner agencies to learn more about the county-wide resources (www.livehealthyfairfax.org/tiles/index/display?alias=chipfeedback)

CASE STUDY 3.1

Setting: Imagine you are a school nurse working in a public middle school. Your school receives federal Title 1 funding because at least 40% of the children are from low-income families. Michael B. is a 13-year-old, Black male student who is well known to you and your staff in the clinic because he comes in often for his asthma self-management. You have watched him grow an entire foot in just the last year. He has always been polite and kind in his interactions with you and the team.

Issue: Today he arrives at your clinic accompanied by School Resource Officer Hollinsworth because Michael has been injured after a fight with another male student in the hallway. Officer Hollinsworth tells Michael that after his injuries, they are headed to the principal's office to initiate an out-of-school suspension. You are concerned by Officer Hollinsworth's words and tone. You are aware of the "school-to-prison pipeline" phenomenon and question Officer Hollinsworth's intentions. You are further concerned because you know Michael's parents both work, and will most likely not be available to come in and advocate for him.

Case Study Questions

What would you do short-term and long-term to help in optimizing Michael's health and learning needs and those of his fellow students?

1. In addition to addressing Michael's physical injury, what other aspects of his health and wellness should you consider? For example, consider conducting a Pediatric ACEs and Related Life-events Screener (PEARLS) assessment and/or one of the social determinants of health screening tools. How might you incorporate this screening into the clinic's practice?
2. How might you ensure Michael has an adult advocate for him during his meeting with the principal and the school resource officer? If you can't leave the clinic, who are other staff or teachers in the school who could help?
3. You are concerned that Michael is being racially targeted. You wonder about the school's racial/ethnic patterns for disciplinary action. How might you approach your principal?
4. What could you do proactively to address bias and discrimination in the school's policies and practices? How might you help promote health equity by establishing a school-district wellness program with your school-based committees?
5. What role might the Parent, Student, Teacher Association play in developing evidence-based antiracism policies and practices such as restorative justice programs (Walker, 2020) and/or school-based health centers with wrap-around (physical, mental, and dental) services? Who might be the other stakeholders in the school and in the community?

REFERENCES

American Association of Family Physicians. (2022). The everyone project toolkit. https://www.aafp.org/family-physician/patient-care/the-everyone-project/toolkit.html

American Public Health Association. (2020, October 24). *Structural racism is a public health crisis: Impact on the black community.* Policy: LB20-04. https://www.apha.org/policies-and-advocacy/public-health-policy-statements/policy-database/2021/01/13/structural-racism-is-a-public-health-crisis

Anderson, K. M. (Ed.). (2012). *How far have we come in reducing health disparities?: Progress since 2000: Workshop summary.* National Academies Press. https://www.nap.edu/read/13383/chapter/1

Anstey, K., & Wright, L. (2014). Responding to discriminatory requests for a different healthcare provider. *Nursing Ethics, 21*(1), 86–96. https://doi.org/10.1177/0969733013486799

The BIPOC Project: A Black, Indigenous, & People of Color Movement. (n.d.). https://www.thebipocproject.org/

Bourgois, P., Holmes, S. M., Sue, K., & Quesada, J. (2017). Structural vulnerability: Operationalizing the concept to address health disparities in clinical care. *Academic Medicine: Journal of the Association of American Medical Colleges, 92*(3), 299–307. https://doi.org/10.1097/ACM.0000000000001294

Bourke, B. (2016). Meaning and implications of being labelled a predominantly white institution. *College and University, 91*(3), 12–18, 20–21. http://proxygw.wrlc.org/login?url=https://www-proquest-com.proxygw.wrlc.org/scholarly-journals/meaning-implications-being-labelled-predominantly/docview/1819910716/se-2?accountid=11243

Brady, J. M. (2014). The racist patient – Revisited. *Journal of Perianesthesia Nursing: Official Journal of the American Society of Perianesthesia Nurses, 29*(3), 239–241. https://doi.org/10.1016/j.jopan.2014.03.008

Brown, C. M., & Dancy, E. T. (2010). Predominantly white institutions. In K. Lomotey (Ed.), *Encyclopedia of African American education* (pp. 524–526). SAGE Publications, Inc., https://www.doi.org/10.4135/9781412971966.n193

California Newsreel. (2008a). When the bough breaks. https://unnaturalcauses.org/assets/uploads/file/UC_Transcript2_annotated.pdf

California Newsreel. (2008b). In sickness and in wealth. https://unnaturalcauses.org/transcripts.php

Centers for Medicare & Medicaid Services. (2020). Accountable communities health model. https://innovation.cms.gov/innovation-models/ahcm

Center on the Developing Child: Harvard University. (n.d.). Take the ACE quiz – And learn what it does and doesn't mean. https://developingchild.harvard.edu/media-coverage/take-the-ace-quiz-and-learn-what-it-does-and-doesnt-mean/

David, E. J. R. (Ed.). (2014). *Internalized oppression: The psychology of marginalized groups.* Springer Publishing Company.

Davis, S. (2022). The National League for Nursing/Walden University College of Nursing Institute for Social Determinants of Health and Social Change. *Nursing Education Perspectives, 43*(1), 68–69.

Falson, J. R. (2020, 24 June). A letter to white people: Black Americans are exhausted. *The Tennessean*. https://www.tennessean.com/story/opinion/2020/06/24/letter-white-people-black-americans-exhausted/3247279001/

Fears, D. (2020, November 16). Shingle mountain. https://www.washingtonpost.com/climate-environment/2020/11/16/environmental-racism-dallas-shingle-mountain/?arc404=true

Felitti, V. J., Anda, R. F., Nordenberg, D., Williamson, D. F., Spitz, A. M., Edwards, V., & Marks, J. S. (1998). Relationship of childhood abuse and household dysfunction to many of the leading causes of death in adults: The Adverse Childhood Experiences (ACE) study. *American Journal of Preventive Medicine, 14*(4), 245–258.

Franklin, J. H., & The Advisory Board to the President's Initiative on Race. (1998, September). One America in the 21st century: Forging a new future: The President's Initiative on Race: The Advisory Board's Report to the President. https://www.ncjrs.gov/txtfiles/173431.txt

Garza, F. (2021, February 11). *America's dirty divide: How environmental racism leaves the vulnerable behind*. https://www.theguardian.com/us-news/2021/feb/11/environmental-racism-americas-dirty-divide

Geronimus, A. T., Hicken, M. T., Pearson, J. A., Seashols, S. J., Brown, K. L., & Cruz, T. D. (2010). Do US black women experience stress-related accelerated biological aging? *Human Nature, 21*(1), 19–38.

Griffith, A. N., Hurd, N. M., & Hussain, S. B. (2019). "I didn't come to school for this": A qualitative examination of experiences with race-related stressors and coping responses among Black students attending a predominantly White institution. *Journal of Adolescent Research, 34*(2), 115–139.

Hansen, H., & Metzl, J. M. (2017). New medicine for the U.S. Health Care System: Training physicians for structural interventions. *Academic Medicine: Journal of the Association of American Medical Colleges, 92*(3), 279–281. https://doi.org/10.1097/ACM.0000000000001542

Holmes, S. L., Ebbers, L. H., Robinson, D. C., & Mugenda, A. G. (2000). Validating African American students at predominantly White institutions. *Journal of College Student Retention: Research, Theory & Practice, 2*(1), 41–58.

Hostetter, M., & Klein, S. (2018). *In focus: Reducing racial disparities in health care by confronting racism*. The Commonwealth Fund. https://www.commonwealthfund.org/publications/2018/sep/focus-reducing-racial-disparities-health-care-confronting-racism

Institute for Healthcare Improvement. (2017). Liberation in the exam room: Racial justice and equity in health care. http://www.ihi.org/resources/Pages/Tools/Liberation-in-the-Exam-Room-Racial-Justice-Equity-in-Health-Care.aspx

Institute of Medicine (US) Committee on Quality of Health Care in America, L. T. Kohn, J. M. Corrigan, & M. S. Donaldson, (Eds.). (2000). *To err is human: Building a safer health system*. National Academies Press (US).

Jones, C. P. (2018). Toward the science and practice of anti-racism: Launching a national campaign against racism. *Ethnicity & Disease, 28*(Suppl 1), 231–234. https://doi.org/10.18865/ed.28.S1.231

Jones, C. P., Jones, C. Y., Perry, G. S., Barclay, G., & Jones, C. A. (2009). Addressing the social determinants of children's health: A cliff analogy. *Journal of Health Care for the Poor and Underserved, 20*(4), 1–12.

Landrine, H., & Corral, I. (2009). Separate and unequal: Residential segregation and black health disparities. *Ethnicity & Disease, 19*(2), 179.

Legha, R. K., Williams, D. R., Snowden, L., & Miranda, J. (2020, November 4). Getting our knees off Black people's necks: An anti-racist approach to medical care. *Health Affairs.* https://doi.org/10.1377/hblog20201029.167296

Live Healthy Fairfax. (2018, December 23). *Community Health Improvement Plan 2019–2023.* http://www.livehealthyfairfax.org/content/sites/fairfax/community-health-improvement-plan-2019-2023.pdf

Love, H. E., Schlitt, J., Soleimanpour, S., Panchal, N., & Behr, C. (2019). Twenty years of school-based health care growth and expansion. *Health Affairs, 38*(5), 755–764.

Lussenhop, J. (2016, April 18). Clinton crime bill: Why is it so controversial? https://www.bbc.com/news/world-us-canada-36020717

Martin, N., & Montagne, R. (2017, December 7). Nothing protects black women from dying in pregnancy and childbirth. *ProPublica.* https://assets.propublica.org/pdf/Lost-Mothers-Black-Women.pdf

Matthew, D. B. (2018). *Just medicine: A cure for racial inequality in American health care.* NYU Press.

Metzl, J. M., & Hansen, H. (2014). Structural competency: Theorizing a new medical engagement with stigma and inequality. *Social Science & Medicine, 103*, 126–133. https://doi.org/10.1016/j.socscimed.2013.06.032

Metzl, J. M., Petty, J., & Olowojoba, O. V. (2018). Using a structural competency framework to teach structural racism in pre-health education. *Social Science & Medicine, 199*, 189–201. https://doi.org/10.1016/j.socscimed.2017.06.029

Michigan Health Council. (2020, August 28). Education series on health equity and implicit bias. https://mhc.org/2020/08/28/michigan-health-council-provides-free-educational-series-to-address-health-equity-and-implicit-bias/

Moore, K. (2020, May 27). Structural racism a public health crisis. https://www.naacpldf.org/naacp-publications/ldf-blog/structural-racism-is-a-public-health-crisis/

National Association of School Nurses. (June, 2020). Position brief – Eliminate racism to optimize student health and learning. https://www.nasn.org/advocacy/professional-practice-documents/positionbriefs/pb-racism

Nelson, L., & Lind, D. (2015, October 27). The school-to-prison pipeline, explained. https://www.vox.com/2015/2/24/8101289/school-discipline-race

O'Gurek, D. T., & Henke, C. (2018). A practical approach to screening for social determinants of health. *Family Practice Management, 25*(3), 7–12. https://www.aafp.org/fpm/2018/0500/p7.html?cmpid=em_FPM_20180516

O'Hara, D. (21 February, 2018). David Williams studies health disparities in America. https://www.apa.org/members/content/williams-health-disparities

The Ohio State Wexner Medical Center. (2020). Anti-racism initiatives. https://wexnermedical.osu.edu/about-us/anti-racism-initiative

Petersen, E. E., Davis, N. L., Goodman, D., Cox, S., Syverson, C., Seed, K., & Barfield, W. (2019). Racial/ethnic disparities in pregnancy-related deaths – United States, 2007–2016. *Morbidity and Mortality Weekly Report, 68*(35), 762.

The PRAPARE Screening Tool. (2022). https://prapare.org/the-prapare-screening-tool/

The Philadelphia ACE Project. (2021). https://www.philadelphiaaces.org/

Purpose Built Communities. (2012, October 1). East Lake went from 'War Zone' to a national model. https://purposebuiltcommunities.org/east-lake-went-from-war-zone-to-a-national-model/

Purpose Built Communities. (2021). https://purposebuiltcommunities.org/

Robert Wood Johnson Foundation (RWJF). (2013). *Metro map.* Infographic. https://www.rwjf.org/en/library/infographics/washington-dc-map.html

Seymour, S., & Ray, J. (2015). Grads of historically black colleges have well-being edge. Gallup.com, 1127. https://hbcufirst.com/Portals/20/Research/news-gallup-com-poll-186362-grads-historically-black-colleges-edge-aspx.pdf

Solar, O., & Irwin, A. (2010). *A conceptual framework for action on the social determinants of health: Social determinants of health discussion paper 2 (Policy and Practice).* World Health Organization.

Tervalon, M., & Murray-Garcia, J. (1998). Cultural humility versus cultural competence: A critical distinction in defining physician training outcomes in multicultural education. *Journal of Health Care for the Poor and Underserved, 9*(2), 117–125.

Tung, E. L., Hampton, D. A., Kolak, M., Rogers, S. O., Yang, J. P., & Peek, M. E. (2019). Race/ethnicity and geographic access to urban trauma care. *JAMA Network Open, 2*(3), e190138. https://doi.org/10.1001/jamanetworkopen.2019.0138

Walker, T. (2020, January 30). Restorative practices in schools work, but can they work better? https://www.nea.org/advocating-for-change/new-from-nea/restorative-practices-schools-work-they-can-work-better

Warshaw, C., Tinnon, E., & Cave, C. (2018, April). Tools for transformation: Becoming accessible, culturally responsive, and trauma-informed organizations: An organizational reflection toolkit. http://www.nationalcenterdvtraumamh.org/wp-content/uploads/2018/04/NCDVTMH_2018_ToolsforTransformation_WarshawTinnonCave.pdf

Wyatt, R., Laderman, M., Botwinick, L., Mate, K., & Whittington, J. (2016). *Achieving health equity: A guide for health care organizations.* Institute for Healthcare Improvement. http://www.ihi.org/resources/Pages/IHIWhitePapers/Achieving-Health-Equity.aspx

4

Theoretical Frameworks to Guide Your Antiracism Practice

"We do not make transformative changes in the way we learn as long as what we learn fits comfortably in our existing frames of reference."

—Mezirow, 1997, (p. 7)

Ethical issues impact every level of healthcare: clinical decision-making; institutional budgets; management of resources; and policy-making. The study of ethics is rooted in the arts and humanities and plays a critical role in nursing practice with regard to social determinants of health and the goal of health equity for all.

After reading this chapter, the reader will be able to:

1. Understand key terms related to ethics, theory, and nursing practice to optimize our intrapersonal and interpersonal dialogues in developing antiracism policies and practice
2. Discuss how selected theories from nursing and other social science disciplines help clinicians build their antiracism practice

In the wake of the COVID-19/Racial Injustice Syndemic (Poteat et al., 2020), health professions students, faculty, and administrators are calling for curricular and institutional change to acknowledge and address anti-Black racism, bias, and discrimination (Smith, 2020; Yale School of Nursing, 2020). For practicing clinicians who might not be connected to an academic setting, what are some strategies for not only building our own antiracism practice, but also creating change in our practice settings and/or professional organizations?

In 1952, Hildegard Peplau wrote,

> In each situation, the readiness of nurses to work for opportunity to think for themselves and to share in the determination of what can be done to meet patient needs…is an important factor in defining nursing and what it can do. (Peplau, 1991, p. 16)

Ironically Peplau's words are perhaps more relevant to nursing today than when she first wrote them as we confront the challenges of antiracism reform and consider how nurses can make change within our individual-level practice and the institutions in which we practice.

We can start by reading and then reflecting on the full American Nurses Association's (ANA, 2016) position statement, "The Nurse's Role in Ethics and Human Rights: Protecting and Promoting Individual Worth, Dignity, and Human Rights in Practice Settings."

Now, let us take a moment to reflect specifically on the document's following belief statement: "The American Nurses Association believes that respect for the inherent dignity, worth, unique attributes, and human rights of all individuals is a fundamental principle" (ANA, 2016, p. 1).

Some questions for us to consider:

1. As the most trusted profession in the United States, how do we nurses reconcile our ethical commitment to valuing the inherent rights of each individual with the decades of evidence demonstrating the "unequal treatment" (Institute of Medicine [IOM] et al., 2003) and persistent racial disparities in healthcare and health outcomes?
2. What are the facilitators and barriers within ourselves and within our institutions that impact nursing's ability to provide care that is "just"?
    a. What must we do to fulfill our ethical duty to "reducing the unfair burden of illness, suffering, and premature death of vulnerable populations resulting from social inequities and institutionalized patterns of social discrimination" (ANA, 2016, p. 3)?
3. Who are some of the most vulnerable populations in our communities and in what ways do we, and our organizations partner with them to reduce racism, bias, and discrimination?

Table 4.1

Key Ethics Terms

Term	Definition
Autonomy	In situations where the person has decision-making capacity, they have the right to make their own decisions
Beneficence/ nonmaleficence	The commitment to provide help/to do no harm
Dignity	"[A]n individual's inherent value and worth and is strongly linked to respect, recognition, self-worth and the possibility to make choices" (World Health Organization, n.d.)
Integrity	To practice in accordance with the nursing profession's code of ethics
Social contract	The agreement that a group of individuals makes as part of living in a shared society
Social justice	The recognition that all persons have a right to equal opportunity and treatment in a society
Values clarification	Both an intrapersonal and interpersonal reflection on values and beliefs

Nurses across all professional settings (clinical, academic, research, and policy) may find it helpful to review Tables 4.1 and 4.2, which define key ethical and practice terms, while they build their antiracism practice and renew their efforts to create a more equitable healthcare system and society.

THEORETICAL FRAMEWORKS TO GUIDE OUR ANTIRACISM PRACTICE

Developing an antiracism practice will be a challenging endeavor, for our practice does not exist in a vacuum. Theoretical frameworks are critical tools to help us understand not only who we are as an individual nurse, but also who we are as part of the collective profession, as a member of a healthcare team/system, and a member of society. For example, theory can help us understand how one develops the knowledge, skills, and abilities (KSAs) to "think for ourselves" and/or develop one's "moral maturity" (Sanderson, 2019, p. 168). Kohlberg's (1971) three major *Stages of Moral Development* can help nurses better understand how to develop *moral maturity*, and why it is critical to our role as an ethical practitioner (Sanderson, 2019).

Table 4.2

Key Practice Terms

Term	Definition
Evidence-based practice	Where the practitioner draws upon findings from research, their clinical experience, and the patient preferences in the development and implementation of the plan of care
Ethics acculturation	A career-long process where the clinician develops ethical sensitivity and moral maturity (Sanderson, 2019)
Ethical sensitivity	Integrity, personal growth, practical wisdom, and effective problem solving on behalf of clients (Weaver et al., 2008)
Moral courage	Having the courage to speak up and take action to protect ethical values (Fahlberg, 2015)
Moral distress	"Ethical unease or disquiet resulting from a situation where a clinician believes they are contributing to avoidable patient or community harm through their involvement in an action, inaction or decision that conflicts with their own values" (Sanderson et al., 2019, p. 207)
Praxis	"Mindful action" where one's practice informs and is informed by theory and research (Rolfe, 2006)
Reflective practice	The process of "meaning-making and purpose management in one's professional life" (Freshwater, 2005, p. 1)
Rights of conscience	A healthcare provider's civil right "to practice their own convictions about right and ethical care" (Sanderson, 2019, p. 168)

According to Kohlberg and Hersch (1977) the three major stages of moral development include the following.

Preconventional Level

- Following the rules of good/bad morality as imposed by a "physical power"
- Acting in response to potential punishment or reward
- Viewing relationships and actions as transactional rather than as representing values of "loyalty, gratitude, or justice" (p. 54)

Conventional Level

- Wanting to show respect for authority, to please and/or help others
- Conforming to established moral order out of a sense of loyalty
- Identifying, justifying, and maintaining the order

Postconventional, Autonomous, or Principled Level

- Developing one's own moral values and principles beyond authority or group identity
- Recognizing that what is "right is defined by the decision of conscience" (p. 55)
- Believing in the principles of justice and a respect for the dignity of all persons

Unfortunately, not all members of society reach "moral maturity" (Mathieson, 2003; Sanderson, 2019). If we reflect back on this chapter's introductory quote by Mezirow (1997), we see a path to moral maturity often requires us to have our ways of thinking and feeling challenged, and to be comfortable with this invariably uncomfortable process.

Essential Facts

The more one experiences situations of "moral conflict" (i.e., situations that challenge our current moral reasoning), the more likely we are to develop "more complex ways of thinking about and resolving such conflicts." (Kohlberg & Hersch, 1977, p. 57)

Now let us further reflect on this moral development process, and consider which level we and our clinical team members are currently situated, and what impact these levels have on how we address issues of racism, bias, and discrimination in healthcare.

- Have you encountered colleagues who place a greater value on their allegiance to team members and/or the organization versus speaking up when they believe something is wrong?
- Are there some clinicians who view our daily practice of care as "us" versus "them" or "different than us" versus "they are us and we are them" and recognize the importance of treating each individual client as deserving of care, dignity, and respect?
- How do these varying levels of moral development impact your practice and the quality of care delivered by your team?

ETHICAL CONSIDERATIONS FOR AN ANTIRACISM PRACTICE

Some of us are very lucky and have colleagues/teammates with a similar ethical sensitivity and moral courage. However, when we work within an organization that does not match our values for dignity, equity, and respect, we risk developing moral distress. For example, Severinsson (2003) found when nurses encounter an ethical issue incongruent with their personal morals and values, they are likely to experience moral stress if they feel alone and/or alienated from their peers or institution. Other research found moral distress both negatively impacts the individual clinician and can lead to negative health and safety outcomes for the clients, healthcare teams, and the system (Fahlberg, 2015; Musto et al., 2015). Working with colleagues (both informally and formally) to develop an antiracism practice and institution not only promotes an individual's and community's rights to quality care, but acts as *self*-care by creating a more meaningful and values-congruent practice for the individual clinician. Thus, our efforts toward developing an antiracism practice must acknowledge the ecosystems or contexts within which we became a nurse and continue to develop our professional nursing practice.

Bronfenbrenner's Social Ecological Framework (1977) visualizes how the ecosystems over the course of our life impact us as individuals and our nursing praxis (Figure 4.1).

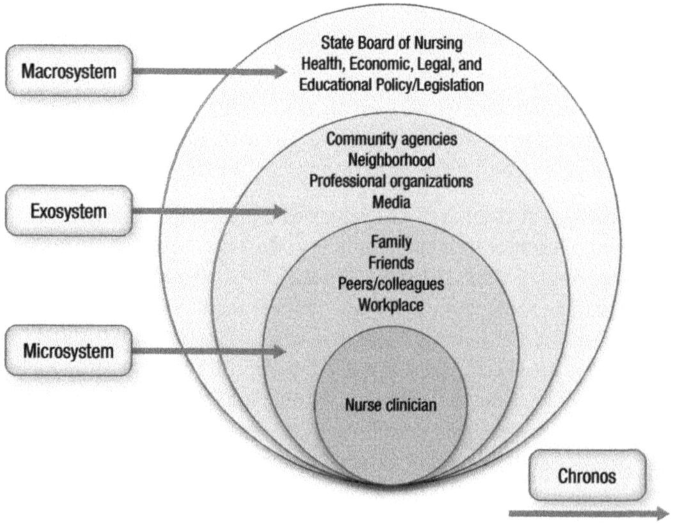

Figure 4.1 Brofenbrenner's Social Ecological Framework.

At the center of the model, the nurse clinician reflects the holism of who we are as an individual. Our status in society is based on our:

- Age/health conditions
- Gender presentation and identity
- Sexuality
- Cultural background (e.g., socioeconomic, religious/spiritual, educational)

The next level is the microsystem, which includes relationships with family members, friends, peers, and colleagues. The level after that contains the neighborhoods where we work and live, the local community agencies/organizations, the professional organizations such as the American Nurses Association or the National Nurses United, and the media in general. In the most distal level, the macrosystem, the nurse clinician is influenced not only by the State Board(s) of Nursing, but also by the health, economic, legal, and educational policies/legislation at the local, state, and federal levels.

Essential Facts

We must take into account that our personal and professional knowledge, skills, and attitudes are impacted not only by our current ecosystem, but also by those ecosystems over our life course.

Several other theories and conceptual models can help inform the development of our antiracism practice. Table 4.3 includes select theories, their key tenets, and some example applications.

A next step toward re-examining and transforming individual-, institutional-, and structural-levels of racism is to develop the art of reflective practice. In the next chapter you will have an opportunity to utilize both theory and reflection in developing your antiracism practice.

Further Suggested Readings/Resources

The Nursing Code of Ethics: Its Value, Its History (Epstein & Turner, 2015)
Foundational and Supplemental Documents on Ethics (ANA, n.d.)
ANA Nursing Social Policy Statement (Chapter: Social Context of Nursing) (ANA, 2010)

Table 4.3

Theories to Guide Our Antiracism Practice

Theory	Key Tenets	Application Examples
Chronic Care Model (Agency for Healthcare Research and Quality, 2002)	▪ Prepared, Proactive Clinical Team ▪ Informed, Engaged Client ▪ Coordinated/Integrated Healthcare System with Clinical Decision Support ▪ Community Services	A nurse works in a hypersegregated part of the city and is caring for a client living with one or more chronic health conditions. The nurse assesses the clients health literacy and then works with the client to identify the structures within the organization and/or community that can facilitate a client's effective health self-management
Mezirow's Transformative Learning Theory (Christie et al., 2015)	▪ Change is made possible from a disorienting dilemma ▪ Self-reflection allows for long-held beliefs and values to be called into question and for new/revised beliefs and values to be considered	A novice nurse is assigned to care for a homeless woman who is diagnosed with severe mental illness and is being treated for alcohol addiction. The nurse soon realizes that the client is a former professor whom they thought "would never" be in this situation. This disorienting dilemma might prompt the nurse to question their long-held beliefs about who is at risk for being homeless or having a mental health condition.
Critical Race Theory (Delgado & Stefancic, 2017)	▪ Race and racism are socially constructed and fluid concepts ▪ Racism is an every day experience for persons of color	Health professionals critically examine who holds power and privilege within their practice setting and in society as part of developing their structural competencies.
John Rawls's "A Theory of Justice" (1971/2009)	▪ Members of a just and fair society work under a hypothetical "veil of ignorance" when deciding on the principles of justice and the allocation of a society's resources	Teams in an organization come together and imagine they are under a veil of ignorance with regard to developing policies regarding requests to change providers based on race.

(continued)

Table 4.3

Theories to Guide Our Antiracism Practice (*continued*)

Theory	Key Tenets	Application Examples
Shearer's Health Empowerment Theory (2009)	▪ Each of us has individual, social, and community strengths from which we can draw to help us achieve our health goals ▪ Empowerment comes from the recognition that we can purposefully participate in our health and well-being	Through the process of reminiscence, we can assist clients/communities in identifying strengths and resources they have used in the past and develop a plan for how to achieve new health goals.
Shonkoff & Garner (2012) Ecobiodevelopmental Framework	▪ Structures/organizations within the child's ecosystem that interact with the child's biology and lead to both short-term and long-term consequences to health and well-being	Consider the disproportionality of school disciplinary policies for students of color and the impact that the school-prison pipeline has on Black and Brown communities.
Leininger's Culture Care: Diversity and Universality Theory (Nursing-theory.org, n.d.)	▪ Nursing is a humanistic profession that works with clients to preserve, accommodate, or repattern the clients' cultural preferences depending on how those preferences impact the clients' health and well-being	A nurse works with colleagues to develop policies and procedures that meet infection control guidelines so that postpartum women can take their placentas home for burial.
Syndemics Model of Health (Singer et al., 2017)	▪ Considers the interaction effects among health conditions and social conditions and their contribution to health inequity	The certified nurse midwife and healthcare team recognize that racism/the "weathering" effect contributes to the higher rates of Black maternal morbidity and mortality.

REFERENCES

Agency for Healthcare Research and Quality. (2013, May). Module 16. Introduction to the care model. https://www.ahrq.gov/ncepcr/tools/pf-handbook/mod16.html#bodenheimer

American Nurses Association. (n.d.). Foundational and supplemental documents. https://www.nursingworld.org/practice-policy/nursing-excellence/ethics/foundational-and-supplemental-documents/

American Nurses Association. (2010). Nursing's social policy statement: The essence of the profession. Nursesbooks.org.

American Nurses Association (ANA). (2016). The nurse's role in ethics and human rights: Protecting and promoting individual worth, dignity, and human rights in practice settings. Retrieved September 2, 2020 from https://www.nursingworld.org/~4af078/globalassets/docs/ana/ethics/ethics-and-human-rights-protecting-and-promoting-final-formatted-20161130.pdf

Bronfenbrenner, U. (1977). Toward an experimental ecology of human development. *American Psychologist, 32*(7), 513.

Christie, M., Carey, M., Robertson, A., & Grainger, P. (2015). Putting transformative learning theory into practice. *Australian Journal of Adult Learning, 55*, 9–30.

Delgado, R., & Stefancic, J. (2017). *Critical race theory: An introduction* (Vol. 20). NYU Press. Retrieved August 29, 2020 from https://static1.squarespace.com/static/5441df7ee4b02f59465d2869/t/5d8e9fdec6720c0557cf55fa/1569628126531/DELGADO++Critical+Race+Theory.pdf

Epstein, B., & Turner, M. (2015). The nursing code of ethics: Its value, its history. *Online Journal of Issues in Nursing, 20*(2), 1–10. https://doi.org/10.3912/OJIN.Vol20No02Man04

Fahlberg, B. (2015). Moral courage: A step beyond patient advocacy. *Nursing, 45*(6), 13–14. https://doi.org/10.1097/01.NURSE.0000464991.63854.51

Freshwater, D. (2005). *Transforming nursing through reflective practice*. Blackwell Publishing.

Institute of Medicine (US) Committee on Understanding and Eliminating Racial and Ethnic Disparities in Health Care, B. D. Smedley, A. Y. Stith, & A. R. Nelson, (Eds.). (2003). *Unequal treatment: Confronting racial and ethnic disparities in health care*. National Academies Press (US). https://doi.org/10.17226/10260.

Kohlberg, L. (1971). Stages of moral development as a basis for moral education. *Moral Education: Interdisciplinary Approaches*, 23–92.

Kohlberg, L., & Hersh, R. H. (1977). Moral development: A review of the theory. *Theory Into Practice, 16*(2), 53–59.

Mathieson, K. (2003). Elements of moral maturity. *Journal of College and Character, 4*(5). https://doi.org/10.2202/1940-1639.1356.

Mezirow, J. (1997). Transformative learning: Theory to practice. *New Directions for Adult and Continuing Education, 1997*(74), 5–12.

Musto, L. C., Rodney, P. A., & Vanderheide, R. (2015). Toward interventions to address moral distress: Navigating structure and agency. *Nursing Ethics, 22*(1), 91–102. https://doi.org/10.1177/0969733014534879.

Nursing-theory.org. (n.d.). Culture care theory. Retrieved September 2, 2020 from: https://nursing-theory.org/theories-and-models/leininger-culture-care-theory.php

Peplau, H. E. (1991). *Interpersonal relations in nursing: A conceptual frame of reference for psychodynamic nursing*. Springer Publishing Company.

Poteat, T., Millett, G. A., Nelson, L. E., & Beyrer, C. (2020). Understanding COVID-19 risks and vulnerabilities among black communities in America: The lethal force of syndemics. *Annals of Epidemiology, 47*, 1–3. https://doi.org/10.1016/j.annepidem.2020.05.004.

Rawls, J. (1971/2009). A theory of justice: Revised edition. Harvard University Press. https://d1wqtxts1xzle7.cloudfront.net/38030445/A_Theory_of_Justice-john_rawls.pdf?1435517838=&response-content-disposition=inline%3B+filename%3DA_THEORY_OF_JUSTICE.pdf&Expires=1609621577&Signature=f2d4An-jsfD~rJMWAvi1gwEtzkmf8fuDVlq50kqXtszx2EnSFiAUSDNBhV9QEpHeAY2IDpOeskHaS9JtrqmfVjxefu9qMuEQ7-vRqSDr7WbL0~kE6NbubCC-oM7V7YgZPk8SKRofQcVXY3FhdjTHFPifbleXMId17b7beOp0GGs84QUCCT0b~1JejMXzuqN-wedDDaJOaOAjAztU4w8HjVHGxfFsVSwguVp5kdbrrCAYRDaZVp1JytlftRqgYMAC-3cyxDP9XFHUzk7O8-hFoCAAd3DKkico5yqzLdHn5Xk~61bhNLhenhj62Dg4n56Vce7vsMWXgfw4TQYwIXzitQ__&Key-Pair-Id=APKAJLOHF5GGSLRBV4ZA

Rolfe, G. (2006). Nursing praxis and the science of the unique. *Nursing Science Quarterly, 19*(1), 39–43.

Sanderson, C. D. (2019) Ethical and bioethical issues in nursing and health care. In B. Cherry & S. R. Jacob (Eds.), *Contemporary Nursing: Issues, Trends, and Management* (8th ed., pp. 161–178). Elsevier.

Sanderson, C., Sheahan, L., Kochovska, S., Luckett, T., Parker, D., Butow, P., & Agar, M. (2019). Re-defining moral distress: A systematic review and critical re-appraisal of the argument-based bioethics literature. *Clinical Ethics, 14*(4), 195–210.

Severinsson, E. (2003). Moral stress and burnout: Qualitative content analysis. *Nursing & Health Sciences, 5*(1), 59–66.

Shearer, N. B. (2009). Health empowerment theory as a guide for practice. *Geriatric Nursing, 30*(2 Suppl), 4–10. https://doi.org/10.1016/j.gerinurse.2009.02.003

Shonkoff, J. P., & Garner, A. S. (2012). Committee on psychosocial aspects of child and family health, committee on early childhood, adoption, and dependent care, & section on developmental and behavioral pediatrics. The lifelong effects of early childhood adversity and toxic stress. *Pediatrics, 129*(1), e232–e246. https://doi.org/10.1542/peds.2011-2663.

Singer, M., Bulled, N., Ostrach, B., & Mendenhall, E. (2017). Syndemics and the biosocial conception of health. *Lancet, 389*(10072), 941–950.

Smith, T. M. (2020, July 28). Ending health inequity requires new skill: structural competency. American Medical Association. https://www.ama-assn.org/education/accelerating-change-medical-education/ending-health-inequity-requires-new-skill

Weaver, K., Morse, J., & Mitcham, C. (2008). Ethical sensitivity in professional practice: Concept analysis. *Journal of Advanced Nursing, 62*(5), 607–618.

World Health Organization. (n.d.). World Mental Health Day 2015: Dignity and mental health information sheet. https://www.who.int/mental_health/world-mental-health-day/infosheet_wmhd2015.pdf?ua=1#:~:text=Dignity%20refers%20to%20an%20individual's,with%20dignity%20stems%20from%20the

Yale School of Nursing. (2020, June 18). YSN announces its commitment to anti-racism [Press Release]. https://nursing.yale.edu/news/ysn-announces-its-commitment-anti-racism

5

Building a Reflective Practice to Address Racism and Bias in the Clinical Setting

"The past is never dead. It's not even past."

—William Faulkner

In 2005, a committee from nursing's honor society, Sigma Theta Tau International (STTI), published a white paper, "The Scholarship of Reflective Practice" encouraging all nurses to develop a practice that includes both the processes of "reflecting-in-action" and "reflecting-on-action" (Freshwater et al., 2005). Both types can help clinicians assess their individual practice as well as the systems within which they work.

After reading this chapter, the reader will be able to:

1. Understand why building a reflective practice reduces individual, institutional, and structural racism
2. Identify strategies for building a reflective practice

ENGAGING IN PRAXIS TO BUILD OUR ANTIRACISM PRACTICE

Many of us in nursing use the word "practice" to describe our work in the profession, yet some might argue that practice does not fully capture the holism of our discipline. Rolfe (2006) helps us to see the critical importance of envisioning our work in the discipline as nursing praxis, that is, the process of "experimenting-in-action" or "reflecting-in-action" (p. 40). He proposed that nurses engage in praxis by:

- Recognizing that nursing is a "science of the unique" where the clinician uses three levels of knowledge (the personal, experiential, and propositional) to inform their practice
- Becoming the reflective practitioner by learning to theorize and reason about one's practice

Essential Facts

Nurses across the discipline (i.e., clinicians, educators, and researchers) are to be viewed as knowledge creators who contribute to the holism of nursing praxis.

Reed (2011) argued all nurses should engage in nursing praxis because in "theorizing, practitioners make sense of their daily lives" (p. 26). Figure 5.1 "Holism of Nursing Praxis" provides a conceptual model of how nurses across the discipline (i.e., clinicians, educators, and researchers) are knowledge creators who contribute to the holism of nursing praxis.

Reflecting-in-Action

Similar to Rolfe's "praxis" or mindful action, reflecting-in-action is when the clinician examines their thoughts and feelings during a clinical encounter with a person/family/community of color. A helpful first step is to acknowledge that we all have biases (Tervalon & Murray-Garcia, 1998). From the chronos (time) and ecosystems over our lifecourse, we have developed patterns of receiving and interpreting information that leads to both preferences and biases. By reflecting-in-action, we become aware that our brain is defaulting to a bias. During this time, we can take a moment to self-talk/correct in a compassionate way.

Step 1: Begin by recognizing our biased thought/stereotype, but then remind ourselves the person/group before us is new to us. Just like ourselves, they are unique. It is not fair or just to predict/ascribe "group" stereotypes to the unique "person(s)" (Narayan, 2019).
Step 2: Be aware of our verbal and nonverbal communication. Being mindful and aware of the present moment facilitates our

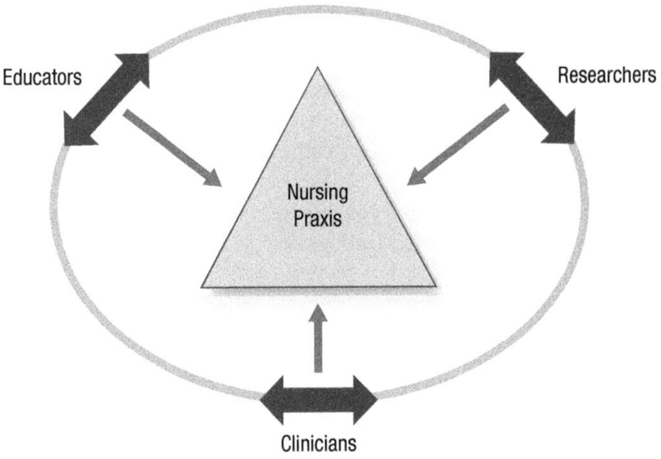

Figure 5.1 The Holism of Nursing Practice.

awareness of these thoughts and feelings and provides an opportunity to self-correct.

- Are we communicating a message of respect and dignity through our words, facial expressions, and/or the tone of our voice to all our clients equally?
- Is the tone of our voice communicating a sense of being ill at ease or disrespect with a client who is different than we are?
- Are we spending more time today in rooms with clients who are more like ourselves than in those who are different?

Step 3: Remember, communication is a two-way process. Our clients and communities also come with their own biases. To foster a trusting and respectful relationship, we must afford them the same understanding and compassion as we gave ourselves when they communicate a biased attitude toward us.

Essential Facts

To help foster a trusting and respectful relationship with our client even when they communicate a biased attitude toward us, we must afford them the same understanding and compassion that we give ourselves.

Imagine you have a racially discordant nurse/client relationship, and the client has just interpreted your distracted manner as stemming from being a racist, instead of from your feelings of being overwhelmed with assignment demands.

- How would you react if they accused you of being racist? Would you be offended and/or become defensive?
- Would you take a moment to breathe and reflect before responding?
- Would you have the moral courage to sit down and frankly acknowledge their feelings and try to correct the misunderstanding?
- What if the roles were reversed and you sensed that a client was racist toward you? How would you feel and how would you respond?

Unfortunately, systemic racism in healthcare is well-documented (Feagin & Bennefield, 2014). Because each situation is unique, it is not possible to address the myriad potential scenarios in this book. A recent article by Paul-Emile et al. (2016), however, offers a "decision-tree" to help clinicians/organizations in situations involving a racist client. Their algorithm takes into consideration:

- The client's health condition
- Their decision-making capacity
- The clinical and ethical reasons for the request
- The potential options for responding to the request
- The impact on the provider

The authors aptly note the importance of Title VII of the Civil Rights Act that protects employees against discrimination in the workplace and encourages institutions to carefully consider each individual case. They also remind us that race-based patient requests are not only "painful" and "degrading" to our BIPOC colleagues but can also lead to moral distress and/or burnout.

Essential Facts

When we feel we cannot continue to care for the client in a professional manner, it is our ethical duty to speak with a manager and find a workable solution that supports the clinician and ensures the client still receives safe, high quality care. (Paul-Emile et al., 2016)

Reflecting-on-Action

More common that the process of "reflecting-in-action," we healthcare professionals engage in the process of "reflecting-on-action" where we re-examine/revisit our clinical encounters and reflect on what went well, what did not go well, and what could we do/create in order to do better next time. Some suggested reflecting-on-action strategies include:

Individual Level

- How did my racial biases impact the quality of the care I gave today to my clients? What assumptions did I make without fully assessing their health literacy or capacity to effectively manage their health?
- Have I and/or one of my colleagues ever had a client ask for another provider because of race? What did I or they do in response?

Institutional Level

- What is our institution's record on patient restraints? Do racial disparities exist?
- What has been our institution's response to patients' and/or visitors' complaints of racism, bias, and/or discrimination?

STRATEGIES FOR BUILDING ANTIRACISM INSTITUTIONAL PRACTICES

In response to the 1964 Civil Rights Act, diversity training in the United States significantly increased (Anand & Winters, 2008). However, in a recent review of the literature, Dobbin and Kalev (2018) found weak evidence to support Diversity, Equity, and Inclusion (DEI)/Implicit Bias Training in the workplace as a stand-alone intervention. They did offer, however, the following suggestions:

- Encourage colleagues to engage in behaviors that expose them to myriad different groups and to create opportunities for building empathy
- Remind everyone that multiculturalism recognizes and celebrates all cultures including the majority group's culture
- Establish a formal leadership mentoring program for aspiring employees of color

Transformational nursing leaders could also consider developing:

- Hospital DEI Committee: Similar to the Ethical Committees and Institutional Review Boards (IRBs), the DEI Committee would review reports of bias and discrimination, and work with staff to develop a response plan.

- Facilitated small groups where colleagues can engage in both self- and organizational-level reflection (Nairn et al., 2012).
- Professional In-Services and Trainings that move beyond "cultural competence," which we still see in nursing (Ozarka San, 2019; Younas, 2020), and more toward a structural competency framework that includes addressing social determinants of health and issues related to racism and trust/distrust. Two excellent toolkits for clinical teams/organizations are:
  - The Protocol for Responding to and Assessing Patients' Assets, Risks, and Experiences (PRAPARE) Implementation and Action Toolkit (2022)
  - Tools for Transformation: Becoming Accessible, Culturally Responsive, and Trauma-Informed Organizations (Warshaw et al., 2018)

REFLECTIVE LEARNING EXERCISE

This reflective exercise can help illustrate how to use Bronfenbrenner's Social Ecological Framework to guide the development of an antiracism practice.

1. Start with the process of "reflecting-on-action" to develop goals and strategies for how you will try "reflecting-in-action." Begin by recognizing that your thoughts and feelings today are a combination of both your personality and your "chronos," that is, your experiences over the lifecourse. To overcome the ego's protective factors, intentionally tell yourself there is "no shame, no blame" as you think about the biases you hold. Instead, act as your own cognitive detective as you reflect on these thoughts and feelings. Journaling or concept mapping might help with this. This process can be difficult as you reflexively examine both the long-held, unquestioned biases or stereotypes that you consciously have and/or, like many of us, the unconscious ones you didn't realize you have.
   a. First, reflect on the beliefs within your own family (parents, siblings, extended family members) about race and racism. Were they discussed or were they not on "the radar?" Do you recall any specific events where racist/bigoted/biased comments were made? Did anyone question these comments? Briefly review these events and reflect on how these experiences within your family might have affected your thoughts and feelings about race and racism both then and now.
   b. Where did you grow up? Were your neighborhood and school diverse or were they mostly homogeneous? Did you have any

friends, classmates, or teachers who were not the same race as you? If so, in what ways did racism or bias impact your thoughts and feelings about these relationships? Did you ever have an experience in your neighborhood or school where you witnessed and/or experienced racism, bias, or discrimination and wanted to say something, but didn't? What might have been the barriers to your saying something? What might have helped you to have the courage to speak up and say something?

   c. What about the laws and policies at the local, state, and federal levels? Did you grow up when "red-lining" was still legal? What impact do you think that had on your schools and neighborhood?
   d. What about the media, the television shows and movies that you grew up watching and the music you grew up listening to? Compare them to what we see today. What has changed and what seems to be the same? What are your preferences around music, art, and media and what life experiences impacted them?

2. Next, think about how your knowledge, beliefs, and actions/choices are situated within the ecosystem of your current practice setting. How does this setting align with your values and beliefs? Have you witnessed, experienced, or engaged in acts of racism, bias, or discrimination?
   a. For example, have you witnessed a situation where a client or colleague, who is a person of color, was treated with less dignity and respect than you would have "normally" seen accorded to those who are White?
   b. When you have first encountered a fellow employee who is a person of color, has your brain automatically ascribed an educational/professional/socioeconomic level of status?
   c. What is the racial makeup of your practice setting and does the racial composition of the leadership/management team reflect that of the organization and the community within which it is situated? What might account for these similarities and/or discordances?
   d. Have you seen or experienced situations where a colleague engages in racial stereotyping or ascribing reasons for a client's health/behavior based on their race?

After completing this exercise, you might experience some strong feelings of shame, sorrow, and/or moral distress. Some points to remember:

1. We are all a product of our life experiences and "practicing authenticity" means having the courage to be vulnerable "during our most soul-searching struggles" (Brown, 2010, p. 64).

2. Within our own practice settings, we may need to proactively identify and/or develop our own supports as we work to strengthen our individual/shared moral courage and determination.
3. "Never believe that a few caring people can't change the world. For, indeed, that's all who ever have" (Margaret Mead Quotes, n.d.).

REFERENCES

Anand, R., & Winters, M. F. (2008). A retrospective view of corporate diversity training from 1964 to the present. *Academy of Management Learning & Education*, *7*(3), 356–372.

Brown, B. (2010). *The gifts of imperfection: Let go of who you think you're supposed to be and embrace who you are*. Simon and Schuster.

Dobbin, F., & Kalev, A. (2018). Why doesn't diversity training work? The challenge for industry and academia. *Anthropology Now*, *10*(2), 48–55.

Faulkner, W. (2011). *Requiem for a nun*. Vintage.

Feagin, J., & Bennefield, Z. (2014). Systemic racism and US health care. *Social Science & Medicine*, *103*, 7–14.

Freshwater, D. (2005). *Transforming nursing through reflective practice*. Blackwell Publishing.

Margaret Mead Quotes. (n.d.). Quotes.net. Retrieved: August 26, 2020, from https://www.quotes.net/quote/6663

Nairn, S., Chambers, D., Thompson, S., McGarry, J., Chambers, K. (2012). Reflexivity and habitus: Opportunities and constraints on transformative learning. *Nursing Philosophy*, *13*(3), 189–201. DOI 10.1111/j.1466-769X.2011.00530.x

Narayan, M. C. (2019). CE: Addressing implicit bias in nursing: A review. *American Journal of Nursing*, *119*(7), 36–43.

Ozkara San, E. (2019). Effect of the diverse standardized patient simulation (DSPS) cultural competence education strategy on nursing students' transcultural self-efficacy perceptions. *Journal of Transcultural Nursing*, *30*(3), 291–302.

Paul-Emile, K., Smith, A. K., Lo, B., & Fernández, A. (2016). Dealing with racist patients. *New England Journal of Medicine*, *374*, 708. https://ir.lawnet.fordham.edu/cgi/viewcontent.cgi?article=1907&context=faculty_scholarship

Reed, P. G. (2011). The spiral path of nursing knowledge. In P.G. Reed & N. B. C. Shearer (Eds.), *Nursing knowledge and theory innovation: Advancing the science of practice* (pp. 1–36). Springer Publishing Company.

Rolfe, G. (2006). Nursing praxis and the science of the unique. *Nursing Science Quarterly*, *19*(1), 39–43.

Tervalon, M., & Murray-Garcia, J. (1998). Cultural humility versus cultural competence: A critical distinction in defining physician training outcomes in multicultural education. *Journal of Health Care for the Poor and Underserved*, *9*(2), 117–125.

The PRAPARE Implementation and Action Toolkit. (2022). https://prapare.org/prapare-toolkit/

Warshaw, C., Tinnon, E., & Cave, C. (2018). *Tools for transformation: Becoming accessible, culturally responsive, and trauma-informed organizations.* National Center on Domestic Violence, Trauma & Mental Health. Retrieved August 4, 2020, from http://www.nationalcenterdvtraumamh.org/wp-content/uploads/2018/04/NCDVTMH_2018_ToolsforTransformation_WarshawTinnonCave.pdf

Younas, A. (2020). Self-awareness: A tool for providing culturally competent care. *Nursing, 50*(2), 61–63. https://doi.org/10.1097/01.NURSE.0000651628.71776.b3

6

Power and Privilege

"I was taught to see racism only in individual acts of meanness, not in invisible systems conferring dominance on my group."

—Peggy McIntosh, 1988 (p. 35)

Over 30 years ago, Peggy McIntosh (1988) sagely noted that the greatest harms of racism were not from the acts committed by individuals, but by policies and decisions made by those leading our institutions and systems. Her quote here calls upon each of us to reflect on how our country's invisible systems *of power and privilege have contributed to racial inequality and distrust. Today, as our country continues to reflect on the pervasive and persistent issues of institutional racism, bias, and discrimination, it is important to examine these two very important concepts of power and privilege.*

After reading this chapter, the reader will be able to:

1. Understand how power and privilege maintain the status quo of White supremacy and institutional racism
2. Learn why institutional racism is a significant cause of inequality in health and wealth in America
3. Learn strategies for dismantling privilege and power imbalances in our workplace, community, and social institutions

Before we delve deeper into these concepts, let us first take a moment to engage in a reflective "pre-test" exercise by reading and reflecting on the current language we hear about racial and social justice.

Please read each of the following phrases and then think about how they might be helpful/not helpful in building your antiracism practice. You might even want to jot down some of your thoughts/feelings about these phrases so you can compare and contrast how some of your perceptions may have changed after reading this chapter.

- "Thought leaders," that is, those identified as experts whom we believe have the answers/vision versus "egalitarians" who believe that all have rights and should be treated with the same consideration as others (Elitism, n.d.)
- "Check your privilege," that is, reflecting on how your social, gender, racial status contributed to your advantage and/or *unearned* successes (Mascolo, 2019)
- "White fragility," that is, the stress/distress that many White Americans experience when discussing the topic of racism (DiAngelo, 2011)
- "Being woke," that is, by educating ourselves about the history of racism in America, we are awakened and can see/understand the inequalities in our society
- "Being an accomplice," that is, moving beyond the role of ally and actively engaging in acts that dismantle systemic racism (Osler, n.d.)

Now let's consider the important concept of power in America: Who has it and how they maintain it.

POWER

Cisney and Morar (2015) explain a key tenet of how those in power maintain their control: "To guarantee its legitimacy, power must produce its own bodies of knowledge, its truths" (p. 1). Now let's think about this statement in light of the previous chapter on America's history of racism. Recognizing that for most of our country's history it has been wealthy White men who have held the power, how has this group's knowledge and truths controlled the narrative learned by each successive American generation? Now, how has this well-established narrative impacted our interpretation of the events unfolding today in America? For example, compare and contrast the "Black Lives Matter" (BLM) movement for "liberty, justice, and freedom" (BLM, 2020) with the counter movement "Blue Lives Matter," which focuses on fallen police officers and pro-police news stories (*The Police Tribune*, 2021). Now consider which of these two groups holds the general right to use coercive force in our society and which one has been disproportionally subjected to aggressive crime control strategies, such as stop-and-frisk and their related consequences, such as the school-to-prison pipeline?

Since its inception, the United States has been described as the "great experiment." Our *Declaration of Independence* makes explicit: "We hold these truths to be self-evident, that all men are created equal, that they are endowed by their Creator with certain unalienable Rights, that among these are Life, Liberty and the pursuit of Happiness" (The U.S. National Archives and Records Administration, 2020). Most of us were taught to believe that our founding fathers envisioned a country where merit not nepotism or one's station or network decided one's success. These men of enlightenment wished to leave behind a system of government run by a monarchy and the privileged few, and instead create a system where democratically elected officials would represent them and their interests. Yet, for centuries Blacks and women were not eligible to vote and even with the passage of several constitutional amendments that made explicit that all citizens are "created equal," governmental policy and practice have still privileged the few. Indeed, access to power in America still greatly depends on two things: money and connections. For example, think about the many fundraising "bundlers" who President Obama awarded with ambassadorships (Center for Public Integrity, 2017). More recently, Lu et al. (2020) reported that while persons of color are nearly 40% of the U.S. population, they only account for less than 20% of those leading some of our country's most powerful sectors (e.g., senators, governors, university presidents, sports team owners, media executives). In the history of the Supreme Court, even with Judge Katanji Brown Jackson's confirmation, the vast majority of the justices have been white males (108 out of 116) and only four have been a person of color (Campisi & Griggs, 2022).

Severs et al. (2016) remind us that if we wish to seek change, we must first truly examine the political representation in the United States and the maintenance of power dynamics in our society. For example, how is it that despite the tremendous inequity between the "haves" and the "have nots," many White Americans still don't vote their own self-interests and instead elect leaders who often create policies and regulations that protect the rich and powerful? A look back at history provides us with some insight: President Lyndon B. Johnson, wryly explained,

> If you can convince the lowest White man he's better than the best colored man, he won't notice you're picking his pocket. Hell, give him somebody to look down on, and he'll empty his pockets for you." (as cited by Moyers, 1988)

Is it really the case that even poor White Americans choose White supremacy over the election of leaders who could be fighting for the common good? Wilkerson's (2020) brilliant book, *Caste*, helps us recognize the pernicious nature of the caste system that leads higher ranked groups to fight to maintain their power over those in the lower ranks. She cites the Swedish economist, Gunnar Myrdal, who in 1944 noted that the focus of the American caste system was to keep "the Negro in his place" (Wilkerson, 2020, p. 24). So how do we fight against our country's caste system that Wilkerson argues is ingrained in our collective DNA?

One solution to is to revisit John Rawls's concept of the "veil of ignorance" with our family, friends, and community members. We could suggest engaging with them in a "thought experiment" where we could pretend that we didn't know how much power and privilege we might have in our respective social standings and then each of us would ask ourselves what the cost/benefit for us would be when living in an unequal society. We could also continue this work on our own by taking a reflective moment to adopt a "veil of ignorance" in our daily professional and civic lives. We could imagine ourselves either at the bottom or the top of the social order and then consider what that would mean for our life, liberty, and pursuit of happiness. Such thought experiments could provide many of us an opportunity to more clearly recognize the inequalities that exist within our country's current "social contract" (Mills, 2000) and then hopefully engage in actions that lead to more just and equal institutions, communities, and American society.

Essential Facts

Benjamin Franklin in his inimitable wit noted, "...when you assemble a number of men to have the advantage of their joint wisdom, you inevitably assemble with those men, all their prejudices, their passions, their errors of opinion, their local interests, and their selfish views." (Forbes Quotes, n.d.)

PRIVILEGE

Before we examine how the privileging of Whiteness in America has contributed to Black health and wealth disparities, let us first review some key terms and then compare/contrast the status quo with the potential for new directions (Table 6.1).

Table 6.1

Social Structures

Social Structures	Status Quo	New Directions
White Supremacy	▪ Economic, political, and social systems that ensure Whites maintain power over other racial/ethnic groups (Merriam-Webster, n.d.) ▪ White America is rightly in charge and maintains power of our local, state, and federal institutions	▪ Recognizing how White supremacy operates and the need to dismantle racial hierarchy ▪ Working with our communities to mentor BIPOC youth in order to create a more diverse set of qualified political candidates
White Centering	▪ Being complicit in the maintenance of White supremacy ▪ Using Whiteness as the "norm" by which all others are viewed/judged/valued	▪ Being an ally for equity and social justice ▪ Benchmarking population-level statistics where the whole is the norm ▪ Embracing humanism which values all as being inherently worthy and deserving of opportunity, dignity, and respect
Tokenism	▪ The act of simply inviting/allowing minority group members into a group, committee, organization without allowing for their participation to make any meaningful impact on issues of bias, racism or discrimination	▪ Being aware of who is in the room, who has the power, position, and voice to speak ▪ Collaborating in our workplace and our communities to ensure that we make explicit our commitment to diversity, equity, and inclusion
Criminal Justice System	▪ Being uninformed about mass incarceration ▪ Complacency with our system of mass incarceration and the disproportionality with BIPOC populations	▪ Being an advocate for criminal justice and corrections reform ▪ Advocate for safe, high quality correctional healthcare
Economic and Health Inequities	▪ Being unaware of unconscious bias and systemic racism ▪ Engaging in color-blind privilege (i.e., success comes from one's own investment and hard work; Gallagher, 2003)	▪ Reflecting and educating ourselves and others using a structural competency framework ▪ Committing to change at the personal, professional, and community levels

(continued)

Table 6.1

Social Structures (*continued*)

Social Structures	Status Quo	New Directions
Internalized Oppression	▪ Living with the physical and mental effects from how your marginalized group is viewed and treated by the dominant group (David et al., 2019) ▪ Experiencing feelings of "alienation, fear, and distrust" (Bailey et al., 2014)	▪ Living with pride and sense of empowerment ▪ Working toward self-affirmation (Jones, 2014)

BIPOC, Black, Indigenous, and People of Color.

For many White Americans, especially those from the working and/or middle class, it may be hard to conceptualize that they are "privileged." Like McIntosh (1988), many White Americans who grew up in the 20th century believed that the Civil Rights Act ensured there were structures in place to protect Black Americans against individuals who engaged in racism. There was a belief that our governmental and social institutions were not racist. The concept of privilege helps us all to more clearly see why there is much work to be done in order to address health and wealth disparities. Nearly 30 years after McIntosh's work, Collins (2018) provides an update and helps White Americans see what "White privilege" really means:

1. **Power of Normal**
   - Where public spaces (e.g., grocery stores treat Whiteness as the norm and create special sections for ethnic foods and/or beauty products)
2. **Power of the Benefit of the Doubt**
   - Who we trust and don't trust or expect in certain social spaces? The privilege of not being targeted in a "stop and frisk"
3. **Power of Accumulated Wealth**
   - Centuries of exclusion from our capitalist system that has led to Black families having much less accumulated/generational wealth

THE HARDEST HIT: BLACK AMERICANS AND INCOME INEQUALITY

For the last 30 years, social scientists, economists, and policymakers have become increasingly concerned about income inequality in America. Indeed, in a recent 2018 report to the United Nations, Special Rappateur Alston presented some staggering statistics about the growing problem of inequality in the United States (see Section 1. The USA):

- Among 29 advanced countries, the United States now ranks 26th for promoting intergenerational equity and sustainability, and 28th for promoting inclusion
- 40% of American adults claim they wouldn't be able to afford a $400 unexpected expense
- 40% of the population lives in poverty, including nearly one in five children
- Despite being the wealthiest nation in the world, it ranks 40th for healthy life expectancy

Alston further remarked, "The United States has the highest income inequality in the Western world, and this can only be made worse by the massive new tax cuts overwhelmingly benefiting the wealthy" (United Nations, 2018, Section 1, paragraph 4). However, while income inequality certainly affects all Americans, please consider this: The net worth of the average African American household is 1/10th the net worth of the average White American household (McIntosh, 2020).

Essential Facts

The combined wealth of the top 12 U.S. billionaires is equivalent to the entire home equity wealth of Black America (17 million Black households). (Hamilton et al., 2020)

A recent interview with Professor Baradaran, author of "The Color of Money: Black Banks and the Racial Wealth Gap" (Public Broadcasting Service [PBS], 2020) provides insights on how the huge Black/White wealth disparity developed over time (Table 6.2).

So what we can do about it? We can work together to create a new paradigm. Instead of there being a privileged "Political Power Machine" that controls our nation's narrative history, laws, and communities, *from the top down*, we move toward a new societal paradigm such as a *smart swarm* where diversity is valued and utilized to the betterment of the organization, community, and humanity (Miller, 2010). We can intentionally work toward championing diversity as a necessary ingredient for success.

Table 6.2

Myths Versus Reality

	Myth	Reality
Equal Opportunity to Live and Work	Freed slaves could now make a living by sharecropping	Indentured servitude: Tenant farming without opportunity to build equity
Equal Access to Credit	Black Americans could get loans for home mortgages and businesses	Through the 1960s there was red-lining: Banks wouldn't guarantee loans in non-White neighborhoods. Black Americans couldn't get credit and were often left to work with predatory lending banks (Mount, 2017). Still see many who are victim to payday loans, subprime, high-interest loans
Equal Opportunity in Housing	Your income/profession determined where you could afford to live	Homeowner Associations (HOAs) and covenants such as the one in Levittown, NY that kept Black Americans out of their communities (Lambert, 1997). Realtors often would not show some houses/neighborhoods to Black Americans (Reed, 2021)
Equal Protections Under the Law	Constitutional Amendments 13, 14, and 15 ensured citizens are treated equally in society: Equal access to social programs and equal opportunity to participate in society	There was a "breach in the social contract": Black Americans have been shut out of many government subsidized programs that gave Whites access to capital

Essential Facts

Why tax laws matter: Inheritance and intergenerational transfer of wealth is the greatest contributor to the Black/White wealth gap (Hamilton & Darity, 2010).

We can also heed the words of the Head of *UN Women*, Ms. Mlambo-Ngcuka (2020), who is calling for more women in decision-making roles to optimize an "inclusive recovery." During the 2020 pandemic, we already witnessed the success of several women leaders (e.g., Iceland, New Zealand, Germany) in their response to COVID-19. So, what can nurses do (both men and women) to foster greater inclusion of women and Black, Indigenous, and People of Color (BIPOC) in leadership roles within our organizations and our society?

In many workplaces, leaders and managers have developed diversity, equity, and inclusion seminars. If these efforts are to be effective, however, they must be based on evidence. Currently we are seeing a backlash to "required" diversity, equity, and inclusion workplace trainings. For example, Dobbin and Kalev (2018) found that required/ordered workplace trainings are not helpful. They did note, however, that work by Plaut et al. (2011) found that White Americans were more likely to endorse diversity efforts when they viewed multiculturalism as part of their own self-concept (i.e., a recognition that they have a culture that is to be valued and shared). Plaut et al. (2011) also found that a person's "need to belong" mediated the relationship such that those with a higher need to belong were less likely to want to work for an organization endorsing multiculturalism, perhaps because they felt excluded. Findings from these studies are important as they help guide our efforts for creating a more diverse and inclusive workplace.

Consider learning about and/or joining:

- The National Association for the Advancement of Colored People (NAACP) and their efforts to create a just and inclusive America for all (https://naacp.org/join-naacp/become-member, NAACP, n.d.)
- The Showing Up for Racial Justice (SURJ, n.d.).: A multiracial movement that is working to dismantle economic injustice, patriarchy, and other systems of oppression and to "build a racially just society" (https://surj.org/about/)

Other personal actions:

- Explore the Teaching Tolerance website (www.tolerance.org)
- Learn more about the history and mission of the National Black Nurses Association (NBNA; https://www.nbna.org/history)
- Partner/ally with the NBNA, which was created in 1971 and represents over 200,000 RNs/LPNs
- Extend the efforts of the *Future of Nursing* reports (Institute of Medicine [IOM], 2010; National Academies of Sciences, Engineering, and Medicine [NASEM], 2021)
    - Advocate for increased access to affordable health professions education

  - Lobby for increased funding for nursing education loan repayment programs
  - Encourage stakeholders (e.g., schools of nursing, healthcare organizations, and public agencies) to develop programs that will ensure we have a nursing workforce that possesses the requisite competencies to assess and address social determinants of health
- Recognize that institutional and structural racism continue to contribute to inequalities between Black and White wealth
  - Mass incarceration and its impact on Black wealth (Looney & Turner, 2018)
  - Education policy that creates separate and unequal schools (Garcia, 2020)

Personal level: Reflect on your family's story and what role did power and privilege play in where you are today?

To help White Americans examine power and privilege at the individual level, author Saad (2020) has developed a 28-day Instagram challenge and now book called, *me and white supremacy.* Her book is "part education, part activation" as she guides White readers to reflect on how White privilege has helped them and their families succeed in America. Brooks (2020) also provides an excellent prompt by sharing her own experiences with the "Silent Curriculum" of nurses, physicians, fellow students who would engage in stereotyping and biased beliefs about their clients of color and no one would call them out. Brooks's (2020) reflections make explicit the harm done and the messaging sent to the learners, the clients, and the ecology of the care system.

If we think about our clients using the Chronic Care Model, we must move beyond the client/provider interaction/relationship and begin looking at power and privilege in our communities.

Who holds power and privilege in our healthcare system? Consider this:

- Most healthcare decisions are made by hospital administrators, insurers, and physicians who are mainly wealthy, well-educated White males
- In 2019, only 6.2% of medical school graduates were Black (American Association of Medical Colleges [AAMC], 2019)
- Women make up 80% of healthcare workforce, but only make up 19% and 4% of CEOs in hospitals and healthcare companies (Bell & Melford, 2018)
- Black Americans are approximately 13% of the U.S. population, but make up 30% of our "direct care workforce" (Campbell, 2018)
- Who are considered the experts in the media (e.g., television, print, radio) when there is a healthcare issue to be addressed?

Professors of Medicine, the American Medical Association, the *Journal of the American Medical Association*, the *New England Journal of Medicine*. When is the last time we heard the American Nurses Association? What about the National Black Nurses Association or the National Nurses United?

- The health care industry spent $660 million on lobbying in 2017, 75% of which was spent by pharmaceuticals/health products, insurance, HMOs, and hospital systems (Public Citizen, 2018)
- The privileging that comes with assumptions made about who is assumed to be the physician, APRN, or PA versus who is the certified nursing assistant (CNA), the patient care technician, the sitter, the unit clerk, or a member of the cleaning staff?

Next think about who has power in your organization? What is the racial composition of healthcare providers compared to the ancillary staff? Who makes team decisions?

We don't want quotas or diversity tokenism. Instead consider Page's (2007) "The Difference" where the organization intentionally hires/promotes for diversity knowing that groups perform best when individuals with different backgrounds and perspectives bring their "diverse toolboxes" to solve complex problems and/or innovate (p. xvii). Therefore, we can try to encourage our teams to be intentional in recruitment efforts and/or selecting members for committees such as ethics or strategic planning.

How can we address the negative effects that come from centuries of White power and privilege?

In our practice settings:

1. Create a formal mentorship program with BIPOC colleagues who are either in school and/or are contemplating a health professions degree. We can provide encouragement and coaching, along with tips for success, but also recognize the importance of "being real" with them and be willing to share our own stories of success and failure.
2. When the group needs to make a decision or take action, instead of the traditional hierarchical "chain of command" decision-making, we could try a new model, "The Circle Way" (2022) which uses a "rotating guardian" to lead the discussion.
3. We could start more informally by creating a "equity" club and then choosing a book, movie, song, poem, or journal article that examines power and privilege. Colleagues could come together to share with each other, in a psychologically safe place, their reactions to the piece. We could consider how this piece relates to the power dynamics in our workplace and then identify possible solutions for correcting power imbalances.

Community level:

- Partner with a local nonprofit hospital on their Community Health Needs Assessment (a requirement of the Affordable Care Act) and see how we can help improve health equity in our community.
- Consider the work of many national banking institutions to close the Black/White wealth gap by investing in affordable housing, loan programs, and small businesses in the Black community. What could each of our organizations do locally to reduce inequities in power and privilege?
- Support efforts by advocacy groups such as Black Futures Lab (2020) that seek to understand what matters to Black voters and then see how we can ally in their efforts. Of particular concern was their most recent report which found that more than one third of the respondents who identified as "LGTBQ" and/or "Under Age 50" felt "not very powerful" or "not powerful at all" that their vote made a positive impact on their community (p. 13).

CONCLUSION

COVID-19 has laid bare the deleterious effects of systemic racism on the Black/White wealth and health gaps in communities throughout America. In a country where power and privilege have become so inextricably linked to wealth, we are now at an inflection point where we all need to recognize our responsibility to not only call out the injustices, but also become allies in the development of policies and practices that ensure equity and social justice for all.

Post-Test: Go back and reflect again on the terms at the beginning of the chapter. Have your feelings changed? Why or why not? What will be your next steps when you hear people discuss these terms? How can you help foster inclusive and respectful conversations?

CASE STUDY

Your team is discussing nominations for leadership in the unit. Perceived as the same power group, membership is mostly White and leaders are all White. Reflecting on this chapter's discussion:

1. What would you do to promote diversity and opportunity among your colleagues of color?

2. What arguments could you make for why your unit will benefit by having a diverse leadership group?
3. Are there leaders within your organization who help champion your efforts?
4. How might you go about ensuring that BIPOC team members felt it was safe to speak up and that the team was ready to hear what they had to say, especially their perspective around issues of racism, bias, and discrimination? Would you have the courage to speak up and be ready to provide needed support?
5. What concerns might you have about challenges to avoiding tokenism in your workplace?

REFERENCES

American Association of Medical Colleges. (2019). Figure 13. Percentage of U.S. medical school graduates by race/ethnicity (alone), academic year 2018–2019. https://www.aamc.org/data-reports/workforce/interactive-data/figure-13-percentage-us-medical-school-graduates-race/ethnicity-alone-academic-year-2018-2019

Bailey, T. K. M., Williams, W. S., & Favors, B. (2014). Internalized racial oppression in the African American community. In *Internalized oppression: The psychology of marginalized groups* (pp. 137–162). Springer.

Bell, K., & Melford, P. (2018). Women CEOs: The path forward for healthcare. https://www.kornferry.com/content/dam/kornferry/docs/article-migration/WomenLeadershipInHealthcare.Jan2019.pdf

Black Futures Lab. (2020, September). Connecting Black voters to political power. https://blackfutureslab.org/wp-content/uploads/2020/10/HIT-BFL-Deck.d2-1.pdf

Black Lives Matter. (2020). https://blacklivesmatter.com/

Brooks, K. C. (2020). A silent curriculum. *JAMA*, *323*(17), 1690–1691. https://doi.org/10.1001/jama.2020.2879

Campbell, S. (2018). Racial disparities in the direct care workforce: Spotlight on Black/African American workers. Research brief. Paraprofessional Healthcare Institute. https://phinational.org/wp-content/uploads/2018/02/Black-Direct-Care-Workers-PHI-2018.pdf

Campisi, J., & Griggs, B. (2022, March 24). Of the 115 supreme court justices in US history, all but 7 have been White men. https://www.cnn.com/2022/03/24/politics/supreme-court-justices-minorities-cec/index.html

Center for Public Integrity. (2017, January 4). Barack Obama's ambassador legacy: Plum postings for big donors. https://publicintegrity.org/politics/barack-obamas-ambassador-legacy-plum-postings-for-big-donors/

Cisney, V. W., & Morar, N. (Eds.). (2015). *Biopower: Foucault and beyond.* University of Chicago Press. https://cupola.gettysburg.edu/books/91/

Collins, C. (2018). What is white privilege really? https://www.tolerance.org/magazine/fall-2018/what-is-white-privilege-really

David, E. J. R., Petalio, J., & Crouch, M. C. (2019). Microaggressions and internalized oppression: Intrapersonal, interpersonal, and institutional impacts of "internalized microaggressions. In *Microaggression theory: Influence and implications* (pp. 121–137). John Wiley & Sons.

DiAngelo, R. (2011). White fragility. *International Journal of Critical Pedagogy, 3*(3), 54–70.

Dobbin, F., & Kalev, A. (2018). Why doesn't diversity training work? The challenge for industry and academia. *Anthropology Now, 10*(2), 48–55.

Elitism. (n.d.). https://philosophyterms.com/elitism/

Forbes Quotes. (n.d.). Thoughts on the business of life. https://www.forbes.com/quotes/1122/

Gallagher, C. A. (2003). Color-blind privilege: The social and political functions of erasing the color line in post race America. *Race, Gender & Class, 10*(4), 22–37. http://www.jstor.org/stable/41675099

Garcia, E. (2020, February 12). Schools are still segregated, and black children are paying a price. https://www.epi.org/publication/schools-are-still-segregated-and-black-children-are-paying-a-price/

Hamilton, D., & Darity, W. (2010). Can 'baby bonds' eliminate the racial wealth gap in putative post-racial America? *Review of Black Political Economy, 37*(3–4), 207–216. https://doi.org/10.1007/s12114-010-9063-1

Hamilton, D., Asante-Muhammad, D., Collins, C., & Ocampo, O. (2020, June 19). White supremacy is the preexisting condition: Eight solutions to ensure economic recovery reduces the racial wealth divide. https://ips-dc.org/white-supremacy-preexisting-condition-eight-solutions-economic-recovery-racial-wealth-divide/

Institute of Medicine. (2010). The future of nursing: Leading change, advancing health. https://books.nap.edu/openbook.php?record_id=12956&page=R1

Jones, J. M. (2014). The middle way: Internalizing, externalizing, and balance in life. In E. J. R. David (Ed.). *Internalized oppression: The psychology of marginalized groups* (pp. 281–291). Springer Publishing Company.

Lambert, B. (1997, December 28). At 50, Levittown contends with its legacy of bias. https://www.nytimes.com/1997/12/28/nyregion/at-50-levittown-contends-with-its-legacy-of-bias.html

Looney, A., & Turner, N. (2018, March). *Work and opportunity before and after incarceration*. Washington, DC: Brookings Institution. https://mykairos.org/docs/conference/Work%20and%20opportunity%20before%20and%20After%20Incarceration.pdf.

Lu, D., Huang, J., Seshagirl, A., Park, H., & Griggs, T. (2020, September 9). Faces of power: 80% are white even as U.S. becomes more diverse. *The New York Times*. https://www.nytimes.com/interactive/2020/09/09/us/powerful-people-race-us.html

Mascolo, M. (2019). The problem with "check your privilege". *Psychology Today.com*. Retrieved October 10, 2020 from https://www.psychologytoday.com/us/blog/values-matter/201908/the-problem-check-your-privilege

McIntosh, K. (2020) Examining the Black-White wealth gap. https://www.brookings.edu/blog/up-front/2020/02/27/examining-the-black-white-wealth-gap/

McIntosh, P. (1988). White privilege: Unpacking the invisible knapsack. https://files.eric.ed.gov/fulltext/ED355141.pdf?utm#page=43

Merriam-Webster. (n.d.). White supremacy. In *Merriam-Webster.com dictionary.* Retrieved October 10, 2020, from https://www.merriam-webster.com/dictionary/white%20supremacy

Miller, P. (2010). *Smart swarm.* HarperCollins.

Mills, C. W. (2000). Race and the social contract tradition. *Social Identities, 6*(4), 441–462.

Mlambo-Ngucka, P. (2020). COVID-19: Women front and centre. https://www.unwomen.org/en/news/stories/2020/3/statement-ed-phumzile-covid-19-women-front-and-centre

Mount, G. E. (2017, December 5). Black banks and the racial wealth gap. https://www.aaihs.org/black-banks-and-the-racial-wealth-gap/

Moyers, B. (1988, November 13). What a real president was like. https://www.washingtonpost.com/archive/opinions/1988/11/13/what-a-real-president-was-like/d483c1be-d0da-43b7-bde6-04e10106ff6c/?utm_term=.bacafc2e3795

National Academies of Sciences, Engineering, and Medicine. (2021). The future of nursing 2020–2030: Charting a path to achieve health equity. The National Academies Press. https://doi. org/10.17226/25982

National Association for the Advancement of Colored People. (n.d.). Become a member. https://naacp.org/join-naacp/become-member

National Black Nurses Association. (2022). https://www.nbna.org/history

Osler J. (n.d.). Opportunities for White people in the fight for racial justice. https://www.whiteaccomplices.org/

Page, S. E. (2007). *The difference: How the power of diversity creates better groups, firms, schools, and societies – New edition.* Princeton University Press.

Plaut, V. C., Garnett, F. G., Buffardi, L. E., & Sanchez-Burks, J. (2011). "What about me?" Perceptions of exclusion and whites' reactions to multiculturalism. *Journal of Personality and Social Psychology, 101*(2), 337–353. https://doi.org/10.1037/a0022832

Public Broadcasting Service. (2020, July 24). The racial wealth gap? It all comes down to black banks. https://www.pbs.org/wnet/chasing-the-dream/stories/the-racial-wealth-gap-it-all-comes-down-to-black-banks/

Public Citizen. (2018). The $660 million hurdle. Retrieved September 22, 2020 from https://www.citizen.org/wp-content/uploads/migration/health-care-lobbying-report.pdf

Reed, D. (2021, September 17). Realtors reckon with race. https://shelterforce.org/2021/09/17/realtors-reckon-with-race/

Saad, L. F. (2020). *Me and white supremacy: Combat racism, change the world, and become a good ancestor.* Sourcebooks, Inc.

Severs, E., Celis, K., & Erzeel, S. (2016). Power, privilege and disadvantage: Intersectionality theory and political representation. *Politics, 36*(4), 346–354.

Showing Up For Racial Justice (SURJ). (n.d.). About. https://surj.org/about/

The Circle Way. (2022). *What is the Circle Way process*? https://www.thecircleway.net/the-process

The Police Tribune. (2021). About the police tribune. https://policetribune.com/about-the-police-tribune/

The United States National Archives and Records Administration. (2020, March 16). The Declaration of Independence: A transcript. https://www.archives.gov/founding-docs/declaration-transcript

United Nations. (2018, June 22). Oral statement by Mr. Philip Alston special rapporteur on extreme poverty and human rights. Retrieved October 22, 2020 from https://www.ohchr.org/EN/NewsEvents/Pages/DisplayNews.aspx?NewsID=23243

Wilkerson, I. (2020). *Caste: The origins of our discontents*. Random House.

7

Intersectionality

"… character is not only structured by the choices we make, but by the range of choices we have to choose from—choices for which individuals alone are not responsible"

—Michael Eric Dyson, 1992

Kimberly Crenshaw (1989) first described "intersectionality" as a theory for understanding the intersection of Black women's unique lived experience with racism and sexism in America. Of note, the concept of intersectionality arose from the Black feminist movement of the 1970s (S. Smith, 2013). Nearly 30 years later in 2017, Crenshaw expanded upon her theory by explaining that, "Intersectionality is a lens through which you can see where power comes and collides, where it interlocks and intersects" (Crenshaw, 2017).

After reading this chapter, the reader will be able to:

1. Discuss the definition and history of intersectionality
2. Reflect on the impact of intersectionality on our life chances and opportunities
3. Explain how consideration of a client's intersectionality can lead to more equitable clinical care and health systems

Essential Facts

Recognizing the intersectionality of our client's social identities (gender, race, class, etc.) helps nurses better understand the barriers and facilitators to our clients' health, wealth, and well-being.

So when we think about who holds power in America and who does not, as well as how bias and discrimination drive inequities in health, wealth, and well-being, then we begin to see how the intersection of our many social identities impacts our life chances and opportunities.

RACE AND GENDER

Important Population Statistics Related to Racial Inequality

	Black	White
Percentage of the U.S. Population	12.8% (58.7% of which live in the South)	60% (35.8% of non-Hispanic Whites live in the South)
College Education	22.6% (women 25% vs. men 19.7%)	36.9% (women 37.3% vs. men 36.5%)
Living at Poverty Level	21.2%	9%
Unemployment Rate	7.7%	3.7%
Private Insurance Coverage	56%	75%

(Office of Minority Health, 2021)

When examining these population statistics, we see the intersectionality on earnings potential and the disparate opportunities for building wealth:

- Black men are approximately half as likely as Whites (either gender) to earn a college degree.
- Black women are two thirds as likely as Whites to earn a college degree.
- Blacks are also more than twice as likely to live in poverty and/or to be unemployed.
- Non-Hispanic White women earn only 79 cents to the dollar of non-Hispanic White males and Black women only earn 63 cents to the dollar compared to the non-Hispanic White male (National Partnership for Women & Families, 2021).

- During the Great Recession, "prime aged" Black men were twice as likely as White men to be unemployed (38% vs. 19%; Bayer & Charles, 2018, p. 30).

Sororicide

During the women's movement of the 1970s, members of different identities (lesbian, Black, single, married) did not hold the same level of power as White women and this led to fracturing and recriminations (L. Smith, 2018). Toni Morrison warned about the risk to progress from this type of sororicide, that is, the "self-sabotage" when women of different classes, race, and sexuality turn against each other and/or willfully ignore others' struggles (1989/2019, p. 58). What could guide us instead is to learn about the rise of Black feminism, including the Combahee River Collective in 1977, where attention was given to the intersecting issues of its racism, sexism, economic oppression, and political power (S. Smith, 2013).

Essential Facts

Sororicide is when women engage in battles within the gender. An example is the "mommy war" between stay-at-home mothers versus working mothers or the economic/class divide between upper-income women versus working-poor women.

How do we avoid the counterproductive divisions such as sororicide and instead join forces with others who are similarly fighting for a more equal and just society? Some excellent suggestions for *collectively* creating spaces of equity and inclusion come from YW Boston (2017):

- Recognize differences.
  - Our overlapping social identities make us each unique; therefore, respect and seek to understand the complexity of the person and their lived experience.
- Analyze the space you occupy.
  - Look to see who is there and who is not represented, and then work to expand inclusion of others in the space.
- Seek other points of view.
  - Be ready to listen, but do not necessarily expect others to *educate* you.
  - Take responsibility to educate yourself: Seek out podcasts, articles, books, movies, and so on, to develop your own foundational knowledge of these lived identities.

- Show up to support others as allies in others' fight for equity and social justice.

Nursing and Intersectionality

For us as nurses, this means committing to reject messaging that tries to divide us and instead work toward opportunities to unite and join forces: Give our attention to what is going on within our organizations and our communities. For example, the COVID-19 pandemic and its related quarantines had a disproportionate effect on women's careers: The U.S. Labor Department reported that in September 2020 women ages 20 years or older were *four times* more likely than men to drop out of the workforce (216,000 vs. 865,000, respectively; Schneider et al., 2020). Black, indigenous, and people of color (BIPOC) women who work in the child care and hospitality sectors were among the hardest hit (Erickson, 2020).

What can we do? We can continue speaking up and demanding support for women's work/life balance and our many social roles as spouse, daughter, mother, employee, and so on, and our own individual needs. We can look within our workplace and within our communities to advocate for social policies that truly help create equity for all. Indeed, we can join author bell hooks in her belief that "feminism is for everyone" (hooks, n.d.). Figure 7.1 helps us to visualize the significance of intersectionality, that is, how our "overlapping" myriad social identities contribute to inequality and disadvantage.

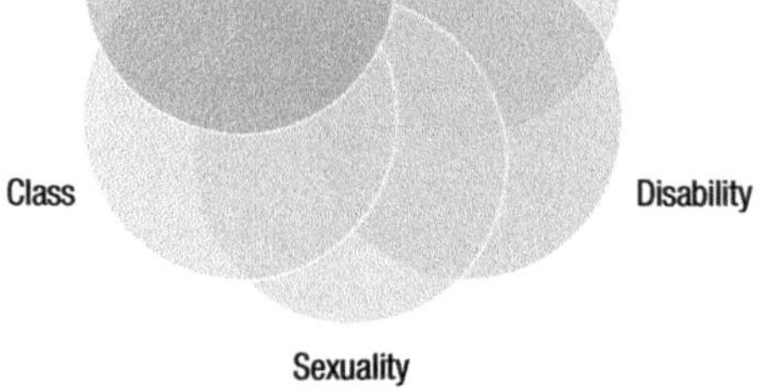

Figure 7.1 The Intersectionality of Social Identities.

Source: Adapted from YW Boston (2017). *What is intersectionality and what does it have to do with me?* https://www.ywboston.org/2017/03/what-is-intersectionality-and-what-does-it-have-to-do-with-me/

RACE AND CLASS

In America, zip code not only plays a critical role in our access to quality housing, schools, jobs, and services, but also "how long and how well people live" (www.countyhealthrankings.org, March 2020, p. 4). Despite decades of federal policies banning discrimination in housing and loan practices, many major metropolitan areas not only have neighborhood segregation by class (income) and race, but also have areas of Black hypersegregation (Massey & Tannen, 2015) and "deserts of disadvantage" (Johnson & Kane, 2018). A recent study by Do et al. (2019) helps clinicians specifically see how the "triple jeopardy" or intersectionality of structural racism, race, and poverty differentially impacts Black Americans' psychological well-being compared to White Americans. The team found the following Black/White differences:

- High neighborhood poverty and segregation led to higher rates of psychological distress for Black Americans.
- Low neighborhood poverty and segregation had no increased effect on Black Americans' mental health.
- White mental health was not affected by segregation, regardless of neighborhood poverty levels.

Findings such as Do et al. (2019) on racial differences with respect to poverty and segregation on health help illustrate how intersectional hierarchies can lead to health disparities and to barriers in achieving health equity for all. These findings also underscore the importance of clinicians considering the role of intersectionality when screening for social and structural determinants of health.

Exhibit 7.1

Universities and hospitals can come together to reduce the cycle of violence in some of our most segregated communities. For example, in St. Louis, Missouri, three research universities and four hospitals created the "Life Outside Violence" initiative. The program offers free case management programs for patients treated for a violent injury (e.g., gunshot, stabbing, blunt trauma). Case managers work with the client and their family for up to a year to help them to learn coping skills and reduce the risk of engaging in retaliation (Life Outside of Violence, n.d.).

Fixing Income/Wealth Inequality Alone Will Not Achieve Racial Equity

How often have you heard comments on Black/White health and wealth disparities like, "Why don't they just…", when the truth is *they do just* and it is still unequal. For example, Mangino (2010) found that when controlling for socioeconomic status, Blacks were more likely to go to college than Whites, and yet a large wealth divide persists. "Informal opportunities" (e.g., greater access to quality neighborhoods, mentors, career networking, informal preferences for White job applicants and/those seeking a bank loan), which are more accessible to those of light skin, help to explain why Whites are more likely to experience a higher return on their investment (Mangino, 2010, p. 164). More recently, Hamilton and Logan (2020) argue that centuries of "wealth generating policies" that disadvantage Black Americans help explain this persistent income/wealth gap.

Essential Facts

Black American families whose heads of household earned a college degree still have only two thirds the wealth of White families whose heads of household are high school dropouts (Hamilton et al., 2015).

RACE AND SEXUALITY

The Human Rights Campaign (HRC, 2019) highlights why it is critical that nurses both assess and address the intersection of race and sexuality on the health and well-being of our African American LGBTQ youth:

- Only 20% of youth reported that they learned safer sex information in school that was relevant to them.
- 59% of these youth reported that their family members "made them feel bad because of their LGBTQ identity" (p. 8).
- Nearly half (46%) reported feeling "critical of their LGBTQ identities" (p. 12).
- A significant majority reported feeling "down or depressed" (80%) and "worthless or hopeless" (71%; p. 16).

HRC (2019) recommends that adults and community members:

- Partner with schools and community organizations to create space and opportunity to highlight the unique needs of Black LGBTQ youth as society often only sees the "White narrative."

- Work with school nurses to examine school policies on diversity, equity, and inclusion and disciplinary practices that perpetuate the "school-to-prison pipeline" (p. 38).
- Check out opportunities to "get involved": Advocate for policies that address the disparities in social determinants of health (e.g., homelessness, juvenile justice, income equality; HRC, n.d.).

RACE, SEXUALITY, AND NATIONALITY

An interdisciplinary organization, the Council on Patient Safety in Women's Health Care (CPSWHC, 2020) provides a role model for creating local, state, and national coalitions committed to providing safe, high quality, inclusive care for all. The CPSWHC's motto on their website reads: "Our work serves a non-exhaustive group of individuals receiving care, including cisgender, transgender, non-binary, and gender non-conforming individuals, transcending the traditional definition of 'women's health.'"

Their organization is part of the Alliance for Innovation on Maternal Health (AIM) that created an excellent Maternal Safety Bundle (American College of Obstetricians and Gynecologists [ACOG], 2016) to help healthcare providers and institutions address peripartum inequities. The "safety bundle" includes strategies for creating:

- Staff training on assessing for race, ethnicity, and primary language;
- Partnerships with community advocates and agencies; and
- Institutional disparities dashboards and multidisciplinary reviews of cases involving severe maternal morbidity and mortality (ACOG, 2016).

RACE, GENDER, SEXUALITY, AND MASS INCARCERATION

According to the Sentencing Project (2020):

- Since 1980, the "number of incarcerated women increased more than 700%."
- "1.2 million women are under the supervision of the criminal justice system."
- "More than 60% of women in state prisons have a child under the age of 18."
- "African American girls (ages 10–17) are more than three times more likely to be incarcerated than their White peers."

Also consider the impact of mass incarceration of women on families and communities. A recent report by the Prison Policy Initiative (Kajstura, 2019) found that:

- 80% of women in jail are mothers.
- Most are the primary caregiver.
- Less than 25% are incarcerated for violent crimes.
- Black women have disproportionately higher rates of incarceration (i.e., they are 13.7% of all women in 2018, but represent 29% of incarcerated women).
- Compared to heterosexual women, lesbian and bisexual women are more likely to receive lengthier sentences.

Of particular concern are the dangers to pregnant women. According to medical anthropologist and OB/GYN, Dr. Carol Sufrin, any incarcerated person who leaves a facility and is considered a flight risk must be shackled (Cohen & Chang, 2018). She argues, however, that these *male-centric incarceration practices* contain inherent dangers:

- Shackling can put a woman at risk for falls.
- Shackling could delay care during an emergency situation such as a placental abruption and/or the emergent need for a cesarean section.

Once out of prison, many recently released women need significant supports in housing and trauma-informed programs as they are more likely to live in poverty, to have low educational attainment, and to be homeless (Sawyer, 2019). While there are several successful "wrap-around services" programs to assist women during their reentry process (e.g., Houston, New York, Los Angeles) the demand is often greater than the capacity (Sawyer, 2019).

Essential Facts

College education programs for incarcerated persons reduce recidivism and benefit society as a whole: Estimates are that for every $1 of taxpayer funds there is a $4 to $5 return on investment (Davis, 2019).

CASE STUDY

This case study can help us put into practice how to reflect on our clients' intersecting social identities and their impact on our clients' and their family members' health and well-being.

Conceptual Frameworks to Guide Your Thinking:

The **Ecobiodevelopmental Framework** takes into consideration the effects that incarceration has on women, their children due to the trauma of incarceration, and the financial costs from the loss of income and the loss of parental caregiving duties.

The **Chronic Care Model** considers the ecosystem in which we live and work. The model helps us as clinicians to remember to think beyond our provider/client relationship and partner with our community institutions and nonprofits.

Setting:

Imagine you are a nurse working on a high risk perinatal unit in an urban academic hospital center. You and your colleague walk into your client's room to engage in the bedside-shift report. As you begin to notice each of your client's "social identities" consider the following questions:

- What assumptions/biases might you and/or your team members have?
- How might they impact the provider/client relationships and treatment plan?
- What assumptions/biases might the client have about your team?
- How might these biases impact the provider/client relationships and the client's engagement in the treatment plan?
    1. 18-year-old G2P1 who is 26 weeks pregnant who has developed gestational diabetes mellitus.
    2. She is African American.
    3. As you get closer to the bed, you notice both her wrists are handcuffed to the bed.

Do you find yourself wanting to know why she is incarcerated? Does the reason impact your feelings about her and/or your concerns about staff safety?

The correctional officer shares that she is considered a violent offender.

So when you hear judgmental comments from yourself or colleagues, you could try sharing Dr. Michael Erik Dyson's quote that reminds us to consider strategies for you, your colleagues, and your community to work together to reimagine systems that promote health equity and community capacity:

"… character is not only structured by the choices we make, but by the range of choices we have to choose from—choices for which individuals alone are not responsible."

Isn't it time to ask what is a better way?

As you reflect on the intersectionality of your client as a Black single teen mother who is:

- Currently in jail;
- Grew up in a hypersegregated "desert of disadvantage"; and
- Has been receiving Medicaid and Temporary Assistance for Needy Families (TANF) services;

what concerns do you have for her and her family's short-term and long-term health and well-being?

Imagine now you are a chief nursing officer or perhaps an elected official and/or a member of a professional nursing association. How might we reimagine the intersection of the healthcare and criminal justice systems in this case study? For example:

1. What if we could creatively design a new system, one in which she could be back in the community, receive high quality prenatal care, and enrolled in the nurse/family partnership or other case management program?
    - With whom could we ally on this endeavor?
    - Who would be the key stakeholders?
    - Who might be opposed to a more humanistic and family-focused system?
2. For the betterment of the individual, the family, and the community, what type of system could we create so that another young woman in a similar situation wouldn't have to be incarcerated?
    - Which the community leaders you might contact?
        i. Try using the Chronic Care Model and then visualize your own potential community partners, such as the superintendent of schools, your school board representative, the director of family and social services, the city/county district attorney's office, or academicians whose program of research focuses on criminal justice reform.
    - Who do you know in these organizations and/or who might help you develop these partnerships?
        i. Who are your local elected officials?

ii. Are there nurse leaders in the public health department you know who might have contacts with the local police, sheriff, and/or adult detention centers?
iii. Are there fellow nurses in your local and state nursing organizations or professional associations who could provide introductions?

- Once you had a team of invested community stakeholders, you might create a local taskforce to conduct a review of the literature, identify successful programs in other jurisdictions, and then collaborate on a grant to fund a pilot project.

CONCLUSION

As we reflect on the complex intersectionality that impacts each of our lived experiences (e.g., self, family, friends, colleagues, clients, community members), let us try to recommit ourselves each day to using our professional knowledge and practice to work toward optimizing health and well-being for all.

REFERENCES

American College of Obstetricians and Gynecologists. (2016). *Safety bundle peripartum and disparities.* https://safehealthcareforeverywoman.org/wp-content/uploads/2017/11/Reduction-of-Peripartum-Disparities-Bundle.pdf

Bayer, P., & Charles, K. K. (2018). Divergent paths: A new perspective on earnings differences between black and white men since 1940. *The Quarterly Journal of Economics, 133*(3), 1459–1501. https://bfi.uchicago.edu/wp-content/uploads/WP_2018-45_0.pdf

Cohen, R. D., & Chang, A. (2018, December 5). *Federal legislation seeks ban on shackling of pregnant inmates.* https://www.npr.org/sections/health-shots/2018/12/05/673757680/federal-legislation-seeks-ban-on-shackling-of-pregnant-inmates

County Health Rankings & Roadmaps. (2020, March). *2020 county health rankings key findings report.* Full Report. https://www.countyhealthrankings.org/ reports/2020-county-health-rankings-key-findings-report

Crenshaw, K. (1989). *Demarginalizing the intersection of race and sex: A Black feminist critique of antidiscrimination doctrine, feminist theory and antiracist politics.* Retrieved October 16, 2020, from: https://chicagounbound.uchicago.edu/cgi/viewcontent.cgi?article=1052&context=uclf

Crenshaw, K. (2017). *Kimberlé Crenshaw on intersectionality, more than two decades later.* Retrieved October 16, 2020, from https://www.law.columbia.edu/pt-br/news/2017/06/kimberle-crenshaw-intersectionality

Davis, L. M. (2019). *Higher education programs in prison: What we know now and what we should focus on going forward. perspective.* Rand Corporation. https://www.rand.org/pubs/perspectives/PE342.html

Do, D. P., Locklar, L., & Florsheim, P. (2019). Triple jeopardy: The joint impact of racial segregation and neighborhood poverty on the mental health of black Americans. *Social Psychiatry and Psychiatric Epidemiology, 54*(5), 533–541. https://doi.org/10.1007/s00127-019-01654-5

Dyson, M. E. (1992). Between apocalypse and redemption: John Singleton's Boyz N the hood. *Cultural Critique, 21*, 121–141. https://www.jstor.org/stable/pdf/1354119.pdf?casa_token=-qd6TTVTdz4AAAAA:5HUhZmdY4yPI5cC792i5qzEdeAROcblyMzWeSo0hdTGtWbZWYa-L7iM8oHBSsK8iQ-EiRnI12WJXz-h_51ys7HlHSDy6DqG7xnkHyuWnFm3zgX-eYsNt

Erickson, L. (2020). *The disproportionate impact of Covid-19 on women of color.* https://swhr.org/the-disproportionate-impact-of-covid-19-on-women-of-color/

Hamilton, D., & Logan, T. (2020, February 8). *This is why the wealth gap between black and white Americans persists.* https://www.fastcompany.com/90461708/why-wealth-equality-remains-out-of-reach-for-black americans?partner=rss&utm_source=twitter.com&utm_medium=social&utm_campaign=rss+fastcompany&utm_content=rss

Hamilton, D., Darity, W., Price, A. E., Sridharan, V., & Tippett, R. (2015). *Umbrellas don't make it rain: Why studying and working hard isn't enough for Black Americans.* The New School. http://www.insightcced.org/wp-content/uploads/2015/08/Umbrellas_Dont_Make_It_Rain_Final.pdf

hooks, b. (n.d.). *Feminism is for everyone.* https://www.plutobooks.com/blog/feminism-is-for-everybody-bell-hooks/

Human Rights Campaign. (2019). *Black & African American Youth Report.* https://www.hrc.org/resources/black-and-african-american-lgbtq-youth-report

Human Rights Campaign. (n.d.). *Get involved.* https://www.hrc.org/get-involved

Johnson, L. T., & Kane, R. J. (2018). Deserts of disadvantage: The diffuse effects of structural disadvantage on violence in urban communities. *Crime & Delinquency, 64*(2), 143–165. https://doi.org/10.1177/0011128716682228

Kajstura, A. (2019, October 29). *Women's mass incarceration: The whole pie 2019.* https://www.prisonpolicy.org/reports/pie2019women.html

Life Outside of Violence. (n.d.). https://publichealth.wustl.edu/gun-violence-initiative/gun-violence-initiative-projects-%e2%80%8elife-outside-of-violence-lov/

Mangino, W. (2010). Race to college: The "reverse gap." *Race and Social Problems, 2*(3-4), 164–178.

Massey, D. S., & Tannen, J. (2015). A research note on trends in black hypersegregation. *Demography, 52*(3), 1025–1034. https://doi.org/10.1007/s13524-015-0381-6

Morrison, T. (1989/2019). Women, race, & memory. In *The source of self regard: Selected essays, speeches and meditations* (pp. 58–63). Knopf. https://theattic.jezebel.com/women-race-and-memory-an-excerpt-from-toni-morrisons-1832540444

National Partnership for Women & Families. (2021, March). *Quantifying America's gender wage gap by race/ethnicity.* https://www.nationalpartnership.org/our-work/resources/economic-justice/fair-pay/quantifying-americas-gender-wage-gap.pdf

Office of Minority Health. (2021, October 12). *Profile: Black/African Americans.* https://minorityhealth.hhs.gov/omh/browse.aspx?lvl=3&lvlid=61

Sawyer, W. (2019, July 19). *Who's helping the 1.9 million women released from prisons and jails each year?* https://www.prisonpolicy.org/blog/2019/07/19/reentry/

Schneider, A., Hsu, A., & Horsley, S. (2020, October 2). *Multiple demands causing women to abandon the workforce.* https://www.npr.org/sections/coronavirus-live-updates/2020/10/02/919517914/enough-already-multiple-demands-causing-women-to-abandon-workforce

Smith, L. (2018, February 21). *When feminism ignored the needs of black women, a mighty force was born.* https://timeline.com/feminism-ignored-black-women-44ee502a3c6

Smith, S. (2013). Black feminism and intersectionality. *International Socialist Review, 91*(11). https://isreview.org/issue/91/black-feminism-and-intersectionality

The Council on Safe Healthcare for Every Woman. (2020). *Purpose.* https://safehealthcareforeverywoman.org/council/about-us/our-history/

The Sentencing Project. (2020, November 24). *Incarcerated women and girls.* https://www.sentencingproject.org/publications/incarcerated-women-and-girls/

YW Boston. (2017). *What is intersectionality and what does it have to do with me?* https://www.ywboston.org/2017/03/what-is-intersectionality-and-what-does-it-have-to-do-with-me/

8

Diversity, Equity, Inclusion, Belonging, and Antiracism

It takes courage to ask—how did I become so well-adjusted to injustice?

—Cornel West

The increasing diversity of the U.S. population and the persistent inequities in health and healthcare underscore the urgent need for a workforce that mirrors the population it serves (National Academies of Science, Engineering, and Medicine [NASEM], 2021). Health equity is the attainment of the highest level of health for all people (Office of Disease Prevention and Health Promotion, 2021). The vision of the Future of Nursing Report 2020–2030 is the achievement of health equity in the United States built on strengthening nursing capacity and expertise (NASEM, 2021). Increasing diversity is essential to meeting the healthcare needs of all people (NASEM, 2021). Along with the increase in diversity is the imperative for inclusion, belonging, and antiracism in teaching and learning environments and practice settings.

After reading this chapter, the reader will be able to:

1. Discuss the history and evolution of diversity, equity, and inclusion
2. Describe how diversity advances health equity
3. Discuss the benefits of diverse clinical and teaching and learning environments
4. Discuss diversity initiatives and best practices

DIVERSITY, EQUITY, INCUSION, AND ANTIRACISM

Diversity initiatives are an integral part of most organizations. Say the word "diversity" and most people will know what it is, or what it means to them, although there is not one agreed upon definition of the concept. Titles such as

- *Diversity*
- *Diversity and Inclusion*
- *Diversity, Equity, and Inclusion*
- *Diversity, Inclusion, and Belonging*

contain nuanced differences; however, they are used interchangeably to describe an organization's mission, strategies, and practices to promote a diverse workforce and foster an inclusive and equitable environment for all members (Mondal, 2020).

Diversity references a broad range of individual, population, and social characteristics, including but not limited to age; sex; race; ethnicity; sexual orientation; gender identity; family structures; geographic locations; national origin; immigrants and refugees; language; physical, functional, and learning abilities; religious beliefs; and socioeconomic status (American Association of Colleges of Nursing [AACN] Position Statement on Diversity, 2017).

Inclusion represents environmental and organizational cultures in which faculty, students, staff, and administrators with diverse characteristics thrive. Inclusive environments require intentionality and embrace differences, not merely tolerate them. Everyone works to ensure that the perspectives and experiences of others are invited, welcomed, acknowledged, and respected in inclusive environments (AACN Position Statement on Diversity, 2017).

Equity is interrelated with diversity and inclusion. Equity is the ability to recognize the differences in the resources or knowledge needed to allow individuals to fully participate in society, including access to higher education, with the goal of overcoming obstacles to ensure fairness (Kranich, 2001). To have equitable systems, all people should be treated fairly, unhampered by artificial barriers, stereotypes, or prejudices (AACN Position Statement on Diversity, 2017).

Justice is related to equity and involves dismantling barriers to resources and opportunities so that all individuals and communities can attain their highest level of health (Braveman et al., 2011).

Belonging is the experience of feeling accepted and valued. It is the desire to have a sense of purpose at work and a sense of community. Garofalo (2019) posits "Diversity is a fact, inclusion is a behavior, but belonging is the emotional outcome that people want in their organization" (Mcgregor, 2019).

Antiracism is the active process of identifying and eliminating racism by changing systems, organizational structures, policies, and practices and attitudes, so that power is redistributed and shared equitably (National Action Committee International Perspectives: Women and Global Solidarity).

Essential Facts

The disproportionate impact of COVID-19 and the tragic murder of George Floyd and others brought to the forefront of America issues of structural racism. America's racial reckoning is demanding that health professionals focus on diversity, equity, inclusion, social justice and antiracism to disrupt structural racism and finally close the gap on unjust and avoidable health disparities and inequities in order to achieve health equity (Davis & O'Brien, 2020; Waite & Nardi, 2021; Whitehead, 1992).

HISTORY AND EVOLUTION OF DIVERSITY, EQUITY, AND INCLUSION

While most organizations believe diversity initiatives are not only socially just and responsible but also morally imperative, diversity initiatives started out of the need for compliance and litigation avoidance (Anand & Winters, 2008). In 1964, Title VII of the Civil Rights Act made it illegal to discriminate in hiring, termination, promotion, compensation, job training, or any other term, condition, or privilege of employment based on race, color, religion, sex, or national origin for employers with more than 15 employees (Anand & Winters, 2008). The enactment of this legislation resulted in a rapid rise in discrimination suits filed with the Equal Employment Opportunity Commission (EEOC). When the EEOC found probable cause for discrimination, a court-ordered mandate was issued for an organization to train all employees in anti-discriminatory behavior (Anand & Winters, 2008). It was not until the late 1980s that organizations recognized the need to transform culture and examine structures, policies, practices, and norms to promote inclusive environments (Anand & Winters, 2008).

In 1990 R. Roosevelt Thomas Jr., known as the father of diversity, wrote a landmark article in the Harvard Business Review *From Affirmative Action to Affirming Diversity* detailing a 10-step plan for creating inclusive corporate cultures, thus pushing past what a single diversity training would accomplish (Brotherton, 2011; Thomas, 1990). He posited that America needed to move beyond (EEO) compliance and litigation avoidance in addressing the challenge of empowering a diverse workforce (Brotherton, 2011). Dr. Roosevelt's model provided the impetus and rationale for companies in the 1990s to embark on training that included social justice, awareness and appreciation of differences, sexual orientation, age, and disabilities (Dishman, 2018).

A similar evolution occurred in higher education. During the 1950s and 1960s in response to federal legislation, colleges and universities started to address the historic exclusion of underrepresented groups from higher education (Williams & Wade-Golden, 2013). Over the past few decades, the focus of diversity has broadened from increasing the compositional diversity of students, faculty, and staff to emphasizing the educational benefits of diversity for all (Williams, 2013). Research has shown that diverse educational environments result in greater productivity, innovation, understanding, intellectual and cognitive skills, and value to the organization (Phillips, 2004; Williams, 2013). The realization of diversity as essential to excellence has led to colleges, schools, and departments establishing their own diversity initiatives (American Association of Colleges of Nursing [AACN] Position Statement on Diversity, 2017; Williams, 2013).

ORGANIZATIONS AND DIVERSITY

The American Association of Colleges and Universities (AAC&U) recommends that advancing diversity, equity and inclusion (DEI), to promote racial and social justice, be a priority for colleges and universities (AAC&U, 2022).

The AACN, recognizes DEI as necessary to:

1. ***Improve the quality of education*** by enhancing the capacity of academic nursing to maximize learning opportunities and experiences for students and faculty alike, which depend in significant ways on learning from individuals with diverse life experiences, perspectives, and backgrounds.
2. ***Address pervasive inequities in healthcare*** by ensuring the preparation of nurses and other healthcare professionals able to meet the needs of all individuals in an increasingly diverse American society.
3. ***Enhance the civic readiness and engagement potential of nursing students*** who will be in positions of leadership in healthcare, as well as in society, more broadly (AACN, 2017).

The National League for Nursing (NLN) believes that diversity and quality healthcare are inseparable and together create increased access and improved heath to eliminate disparities. The NLN remains committed to leading diversity and inclusion efforts that advance the health of our nation and the global community to sustain a more diverse workforce that fosters inclusive environments. In 2016, the NLN created a Vision Series Statement on Achieving Diversity and Meaningful Inclusion in Nursing Education. While diversity encourages self-awareness and respect for all persons by embracing and celebrating the richness of each individual, diversity also encompasses organizational, institutional, and system-wide behaviors in nursing, nursing education, and healthcare (NLN Vision Series, 2016).

INITIATIVES AND DIVERSITY

Diversity initiatives have been around for 60 years, and the demand for DEI is increasing. Diversity initiatives are necessary due to the intractable societal inequities and injustices such as racism, oppression, discrimination, and stigmatization.

Essential Facts

Diversity initiatives should be mission driven. Diversity should not be an add-on or adjunct; it must be central or core to the organization's mission, vision, and strategic plan. To be sustainable, diversity initiatives must have the strong support of leadership. Leaders must be deliberate and intentional in their strategies to create, maintain, and manage DEI within the organization.

For years, through its initiatives, the National League for Nursing has addressed the need for nursing education to step up and lead the efforts to expand diversity among faculty and students. In 2021 the NLN addressed increasing diversity and leadership through its NLN/Johnson and Johnson Project Transitioning Senior Nursing Students in Historically Black Colleges and Universities into Clinical Practice (Brewington & Davis, 2022). Workforce diversity is a key strategy in achieving health equity by increasing access and decreasing disparities. In 2021, the NLN launched the Taking Aim Initiative to address structural racism, diversity, equity, inclusion, implicit bas, and social justice. The initiative raises awareness with nurse educators of societal inequities and the destructive impact of structural racism on access to and delivery of quality care to communities of color (NLN Taking Aim, 2021). The NLN/Walden University College of Nursing Institute for Social Determinants of Health and Social Change focuses on developing leaders and catalysts for social change to transform social determinants of health and social change by addressing the impact of factors such as structural racism, socioeconomic status, environment, education, adequate housing and food insecurity on health and well-being (Davis, 2022).

Inclusive Excellence

Colleges and universities are now adopting an inclusive excellence model for integrating diversity efforts and positioning diversity at the core of institutional functioning. The Inclusive Excellence Model was designed to help organizations:

- Integrate their diversity and quality efforts
- Situate this work at the core of institutional functioning
- Realize the educational benefits available to students and to the institution when this integration is done well and is sustained over time (Williams et al., 2005)

Inclusive excellence consists of four components:

1. A focus on student intellectual and social development
2. A purposeful development and utilization of organizational resources to enhance student learning
3. Attention to the cultural differences learners bring to the educational experience and that enhance the enterprise
4. A welcoming community that engages all of its diversity in the service of student and organizational learning (Williams et al., 2005)

Educational Benefits of a Diverse Learning Environment

- Students and faculty are introduced to more issues and perspectives: knowledge, strategies, applications
- Students are more willing to examine and re-examine their personal perspectives and values; learn more about themselves
- Students are exposed to ideas and points of view that they disagree with or do not understand in a safe environment
- Students and faculty gain a clearer idea of how cultures process the same information in different ways
- Students learn ways of reshaping issues, new ways of reading classroom material, new learning strategies, and are more creative in their approach to learning in general

- Students learn and come up with new research topics
- Students learn and practice new ways of collaborating in class
- Students gain an increased capacity for respect and concern for others
- Students' stereotypes about important issues are more often confronted
- Students' social and political stereotypes are more often confronted

(Kansas State University, 2018)

Organizational Benefits of Diversity

1. Teams are more productive
2. Greater opportunity for personal and professional growth
3. Improves cognitive skills and critical thinking
4. Promotes creativity
5. Drives Innovation

Reynolds, 2021

Equity-Minded Leadership

Leaders are committed to eliminating structural racism by promoting high quality institutional practices that result in deep, meaningful, and lasting change to policies, practices, and structures that promote and uphold inequity (Kezar et al., 2021; Felix et al., 2015).

BEST PRACTICES: MEASURING THE SUCCESS OF DIVERSITY, EQUITY, INCLUSION, AND ANTIRACISM

- Student and employee attrition rates
- Climate Surveys and Equity Audits
  - Workforce and student satisfaction
  - Work place and teaching and learning environments
  - Perceptions of inclusion, belonging, equity, justice, and antiracism
- External awards and recognition for DEI and antiracism efforts
- Set goals, performance indicators, and benchmarks
- Affinity groups
- Pathway programs
- Mentoring and sponsorship
- Retention
- Recruitment

- Admissions
  - Holistic review
- Promotion/tenure processes
- Hiring policies and processes
- Turnover
- Compensation analysis
- Diversity among suppliers and vendors
- Examine and update policies
  - How is racism showing up and operating
- Student and workforce representation at all levels
- Research and scholarship opportunities and funding
- Professional development
  - Faculty development
  - Leadership development
  - Continuing education
- Partnerships - community, academic, industry, practice
- Curriculum development - social and structural determinants of health, social justice, antiracism, health equity

BCG, 2022; White, 2020

All those involved in nursing education—administrators, faculty, accreditors and students—need to understand that health equity is a core component of nursing (2021 NAM Report). Structural racism is an obstacle to health equity (CDC, 2021). Dismantling structural racism and advancing health equity requires a commitment to anti-racism by actively listening, learning, and leading change at personal, team, departmental, institutional, and systemic levels with care, compassion, courage, and empathy.

CASE STUDY

Jillian is a registered nurse on the neurology unit for a suburban community hospital. The unit has several practice committees with active participation. When Jillian proposed a Diversity, Equity, and Inclusion committee the unit manager said, "I do not think we need that on this unit. We all seem to be getting along just fine."

Case Study Question

1. What are your reactions to the unit manager's response?

2. Leaders must be accountable, or risk being perceived as lacking a true commitment to building diverse organizations with cultures of belonging and inclusivity (Corley, 2020). As a leader, can you recall a time when missed an opportunity to advance DEI? What did you learn? Discuss a time when you were intentional in your efforts to promote DEI and antiracism.
3. Leaders must be accountable for investing in their own DEI learning and growth (Corley, 2020). As a leader, how are you increasing your knowledge and skills for advanceing DEI and dismantling structural racism?

REFERENCES

AACN Position Statement on Diversity. (2017). https://www.aacnnursing.org/News-Information/Position-Statements-White-Papers/Diversity

Anand, R., & Winters, M.-F. (2008). A retrospective view of corporate diversity training from 164 to the present. *Academy of Management Learning & Education*, *7*(3), 356–372.

Association of American Colleges & Universities. (2022). *Diversity, equity, & inclusive excellence.* https://www.aacu.org/priorities/advancing-diversity-equity-and-inclusion

BCG (2022). Measuring diversity and inclusion. Retrieved on August 17, 2021, from https://www.bcg.com/capabilities/diversity-inclusion/measuring-diversity-equity-inclusion

Braveman, P. A., Kumanyika, S., Fielding, J., Laveist, T., Borrell, L. N., & Manderscheid, R. (2011). Health disparities and health equity: The issue is justice. *American Journal of Public Health, 101*(Suppl 1), S149–155.

Brewington, J., & Davis, S. (2022). National League for Nursing/Johnson & Johnson project: Transioning senior nursing students in historically Black colleges and universities into clinical practice. *Nursing Education Perspectives*, *38*(3), 140–141.

Brotherton, P. (2011, May 1). R. Roosevelt Thomas, Jr. https://www.td.org/magazines/td-magazine/r-roosevelt-thomas-jr

Centers for Disease Control and Prevention (CDC). (2021, November 24). Racism and health. Health Equity. https://www.cdc.gov/healthequity/racism-disparities/index.html

Corley, T. (2020). Creating accountability for inclusive, responsive leadership. *SHRM.* https://www.shrm.org/executive/resources/people-strategy-journal/winter2020/Pages/corley-feature.aspx

Davis, S. (2022). The National League for Nursing/Walden Uversity College of Nursing Institute for Social Determinants of Health and Social Change. *Nursing Education Perspectives*, *43*(1), 68–69.

Dishman, L. (2018, June 4). A brief history of diversity training. https://www.fastcompany.com/40579246/a-brief-history-of-diversity-training

Felix, E.R., Bensimon, E. M., Hanson, D., Gray, J., Klingsmith, L. (2015). Developing Agency for Equity-Minded Change. New Directions for Community Colleges, 172, 25–42.

Kansas State University. (2018, May 27). The Tilford Group. What are the educational benefits of a diverse learning environment? Retrieved on August 17, 2021, from https://tilford.k-state.edu/resources/educational-benefits-of-diversity/Whataretheeducationalbenefitsofadiverselearningenvironment.html

Kezar, A., Holcombe, E., Vigil, D., Dizon, P. M. (2021). Shared equity leadership: Making equity everyone's work. Washington , DC: American Council on Educaton; los Angeles: University of Southern California, Pullias Center for Higher Education.

Kranch, N. (Ed.). (2001). *Libraries and democracy: The cornerstone of liberty.* Chicago, IL: American Library Association.

McGregor, J. (2019, December 30). First there was diversity. Then inclusion, Now HR wants everyone to feel like they belong. https://www.washingtonpost.com/business/2019/12/30/first-there-was-diversity-then-inclusion-now-hr-wants-everyone-feel-like-they-belong/

Mondal, S. (2020, November 1). Diversity and inclusion: A complete guide for HR professionals. *Ideal.* https://ideal.com/diversity-and-Inclusion/

National Academies of Sciences, Engineering, and Medicine. 2021. *The Future of Nursing 2020-2030: Charting a Path to Achieve Health Equity.* Washington, DC: The National Academies.

National Action Committee International Perspectives: Women and Global Solidarity. Retrieved August 16, 2021, from http://www.aclrc.com/antiracism

National League for Nursing Vision Series (2016). http://www.nln.org/docs/default-source/about/vision-statement-achieving-diversity.pdf?sfvrsn=2

National League for Nursing Taking Aim (2021). https://www.nlntakingaimdei.org/

Office of Disease Prevention and Health Promotion. (2020). Healthy People 2020. Retrieved August 16, 2021, from https://www.healthypeople.gov/2020/about/foundation-health-measures/Disparities

Phillips, K. W. (2018, September 18). How diversity makes us smarter. *Greater Good Magazine.* https://greatergood.berkeley.edu/article/item/how_diversity_makes_us_smarter

Reynolds, K. (2019). 13 benefits and challenges of cultural diversity in the workplace. *Hult International Business School.* https://www.hult.edu/blog/benefits-challengesculturaldiversity-workplace/

Thomas, Jr. R. R. (1990). From affirmative action to affirming diversity. *Harvard Business Review.* https://hbr.org/1990/03/from-affirmative-action-to-affirming-diversity

Waite, R., & Nardi, D. (2021). Understanding racism as a historical trauma that remains today: Implication for the nursing profession. *Creative Health Care Management, 27*(1), 19–24.

White, J. D. (2020, May-June). How to build an anti-racist company. Harvard Business Review https://hbr.org/2022/05/how-to-build-an-anti-racist-company

Whitehead, M. (1992). The concepts and principles of equity and health. *International Journal of Health Services. 22*(3), 429–445.

Williams, D. A. (2013). *Strategic diversity leadership: Activating change and transformation in higher education.* Stylus Publishing Press.

Williams, D. A., & Wade-Golden, K. (2013). *The chief diversity officer: Strategy, structure, and change management.* Stylus Publishing Press.

Williams, D., Berger, J., & McClendon, S. (2005). *Toward a model of inclusive excellence and change in higher education.* Association of American Colleges and Universities.

9

Implicit Bias

It is easy to believe that there is more going on in people's minds than they say; it is not easy to believe that there is more going on in my mind than I say.

— Nosek, Hawkins, and Frazier, 2011

Health equity is the attainment of the highest level of health for all groups of people. Achievement of health equity begins with eliminating disparities and inequities in health care. The elimination of health disparities and inequities necessitates addressing and disrupting racism, bias, and discrimination.

Most healthcare providers believe they treat all patients equally and fairly. However, our implicit biases get in the way and derail our most earnest commitments to equity and fairness (Kirwan Institute, 2018). The persistent, pervasive, and avoidable inequities in healthcare demand that we give serious attention to our implicit bases and their effects in healthcare (Whitehead & Dahlgren, 2006).

After reading this chapter, the reader will be able to:

1. Explain unconscious bias and how it differs from conscious biases
2. Discuss how implicit bias manifests in health care and contributes to treatment disparities and inequities
3. Examine implicit bias formation and how it operates in the clinical setting
4. Discuss strategies to mitigate implicit biases

Implicit bias refers to attitudes and stereotypes that affect perception, judgment, and actions without our awareness (Kirwan Institute, 2018). They are triggered, rapid, automatic mental associations we make and stereotypes we hold about certain people (Kirwan Institute, 2018).

Implicit bias was conceptualized by Anthony Greenwald and Mahzarin Banaji in 1995 (Greenwald & Banaji, 1995). Their seminal paper, "Implicit Social Cognition: Attitudes, Self-Esteem, and Stereotypes," described the term *implicit social cognition* for cognitive processes occurring outside of conscious awareness or conscious control in relation to social psychological constructs: attitudes, stereotypes, and self-concepts (Greenwald & Banaji, 1995). They define *implicit attitudes* as "introspectively unidentified (or inaccurately identified) traces of past experience that mediate favorable or unfavorable feeling, thought, or action toward social objects," and *implicit memory* as influences of past experience on later performance, in the absence of conscious memory for the earlier experience (Greenwald & Banaji, 1995).

The Implicit Association Test (IAT) was introduced into the scientific literature in 1998 to explore people's implicit biases (Greenwald et al., 1998). Project implicit was founded in 1998 by Anthony Greenwald, Mahzarin Banaji and Brian Nosek; the IAT test, can be found on Project Implicit's educational website. The IAT has been taken online millions of times since its creation. There are numerous versions, looking at biases such as race, religion, sexual orientation, ethnicity, age, weight, disability, and an election version that measures unspoken support for U.S. presidential candidates.

The IAT measures the strength of associations between concepts with the point being that responding is easier when closely related items share the same response key (Greenwald et al., 1998). Because users must respond to these pairings within milliseconds, the IAT measures responses that normally cannot be consciously controlled (Greenwald et al., 1998). Test takers quickly categorize images and words as they flash on the screen. When asked to combine words and images that might seem discordant–for example, a picture of a "hornet" and the word "pleasure"–there is often a delay in response time (Greenwald et al., 1998).

That delay is an indicator of implicit bias. Moreover, these biases persist even when the user knows what is being tested (Scientific American Frontiers, 2015).

When the same approach was used to test racial bias with Black and White faces, there was an automatic preference for White relative to Black (Nosek et al., 2002). Frequently asked questions on the Project Implicit website reveal that most White respondents show an implicit preference for White people (Project Implicit, 2011). About a third of Black participants show an implicit preference for White people relative to Black people (Project Implicit, 2011). Asian participants show an implicit preference for White people relative to Black people (Project Implicit, 2011). The IAT might reflect what is learned from a culture that does not regard Black people as highly as White people. Implicit preferences for White people most likely reflect the strong negative associations with Black people in American society (Project Implicit, 2011). There is a long history of racism in the United States, and Black people are often portrayed negatively in the media (Project Implicit, 2011).

Implicit biases have real effects on behavior (Greenwald & Krieger, 2006; Ziegert & Hanges, 2005). There is research to suggest that we act more in accordance with our implicitly held attitudes than our explicitly held or stated attitudes (Ziegert & Hanges, 2005). *This is why implicit biases matter.* Implicit associations are outside of conscious awareness and therefore do not necessarily align with our declared beliefs and expressly held beliefs and values (Ziegert & Hanges, 2005).

The founders of Project Implicit have all openly discussed their experiences with first uncovering their own implicit racial biases when developing the test (Mason, 2020; Scientific American Frontiers, 2015). Banaji describes it as both humbling and humiliating because *you come face to face with the fact that you are not the person you thought you were* (*Morning Edition*, 2016). Everyone has implicit biases. Therefore, there should be a no shame/no blame approach to owning, addressing, and mitigating implicit biases (Scientific American Frontiers, 2015).

Essential Facts

In a study of Black cancer patients and their non-Black physicians, providers high in implicit bias were less supportive of and spent less time with their patients than providers low in implicit bias. Black patients viewed high implicit-bias physicians as less patient-centered, had more difficulty remembering what their providers told them, had less confidence in their treatment plans, and thought it would be more difficult to follow recommended treatments (Penner et al., 2016).

IMPLICIT BIAS IN HEALTHCARE

In 2003, Unequal Treatment, a report from the then Institute of Medicine (now National Academies) concluded that even when access-to-care barriers such as insurance and family income were controlled, racially and ethnically diverse populations received worse healthcare, and that both explicit and implicit bias were potential contributors (Smedley et al., 2003). Since that time studies have demonstrated that healthcare providers have implicit bias in terms of positive attitudes toward Whites and negative attitudes toward Blacks (Green et al., 2007; Hall et al., 2015; Penner et al., 2016; Schulman et al., 1999). Implicit bias contributes to health disparities for Blacks (Chapman et al., 2013; Hall et al., 2015).

Dayna Bowen Matthews in her book *Just Medicine: A Cure for Racial Inequality in American Health Care* states *Implicit Bias, that is unconscious and unintentional racism, is the single most important determinant of health and healthcare disparities and has yet to be seriously confronted* (Matthew, 2015, cover page). Healthcare professionals exhibit the same levels of implicit bias as the wider population (FitzGerald & Hurst 2017; Matthew, 2015). The healthcare profession needs to address the role of implicit biases in healthcare disparities (Chapman et al., 2013; Penner et al., 2016).

Alexander Green et al. conducted one of the most compelling studies to date to address this issue. This 2007, landmark study, *Implicit Bias Among Physicians and Its Prediction of Thrombolysis Decisions for Black and White Patients,* combined the IAT and a method measuring the quality of treatment. Physicians reported no explicit preference for White versus Black patients or differences in perceived cooperativeness. However, IATs revealed implicit preferences for White Americans and implicit stereotypes of Black Americans as less cooperative with medical procedures, and generally less cooperative. As physicians' implicit bias favoring Whites increased, so did their likelihood of treating White patients and not treating Black patients with thrombolysis. The predictive validity of this study represents the first evidence of implicit race bias among physicians, its dissociation from explicit bias, and its predictive validity (Green et al., 2007). Results suggest that physicians' unconscious biases may contribute to racial and ethnic disparities in the use of medical procedures such as thrombolysis for myocardial infarction (Green et al., 2007).

Essential Facts

EXPLICIT Versus IMPLICIT BIAS

Explicit	Implicit
Voluntary	Involuntary
Aware	Unaware
Intentional	Unintentional

Source: Kirwan Institute. (2018). *Implicit bias module series.* Kirwan institute for the Study of Race and Ethnicity. Retrieved May 5, 2021, from http://kirwaninstitute.osu.edu/implicit-bias-training/.

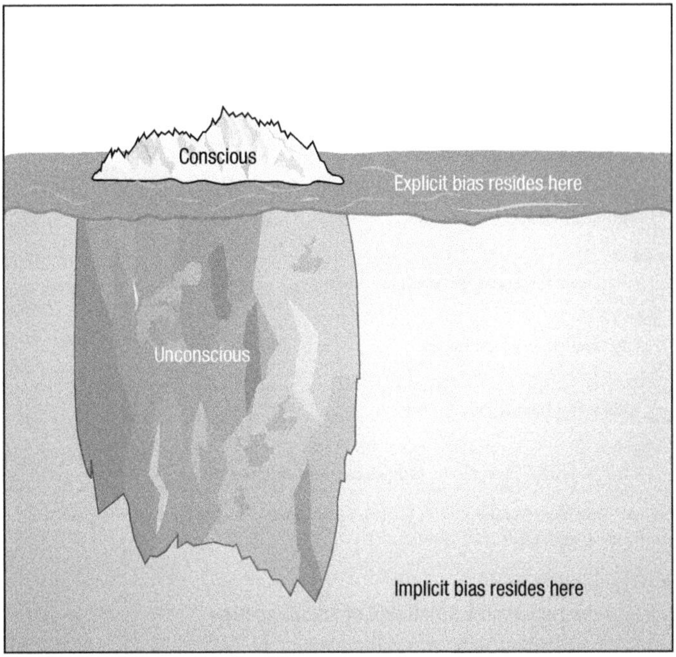

Figure 9.1 The iceberg example.

HOW IMPLICIT BIAS IS FORMED

It is possible to form unconscious or implicit biases based on inaccurate information or stereotypes (Kirwan Institute, 2018). By just seeing concepts grouped together repeatedly we can internalize associations that are distorted and false (Kirwan Institute, 2018). Understanding how implicit biases work in the subconscious mind is foundational to appreciating how our conscious commitments to fairness and equity can be disrupted even when people have the best intentions (Kirwan Institute, 2018). We must comprehend how implicit biases have a profound impact on how we think about and act toward racially and ethnically diverse groups (Table 9.1).

Matthew (2015), in her book *Just Medicine: A Cure for Racial Inequality in American Health Care* provides a schematic description of how implicit biases both form and inform our perceptions, judgments, and behaviors without any conscious awareness.

Table 9.1

Formation of Implicit Biases: How It Works
Step 1 • Store Social Knowledge of Social Groups
Step 2 • Identify Group Membership
Step 3 • Retrieve Triggered Stereotypes
Step 4 • Activating Implicit Biases
Step 5 • Forming Biased Perceptions
Step 6 • Influencing Perceptions, Judgments, and Actions

Source: Data from Matthew, D. B. (2015). *Just medicine: A cure for racial inequality in American Health Care*. NYU Press.

- The First Step
  - Storing social knowledge of social groups
    - This happens over a lifetime
    - What we see, feel, hear, experience in the world around us
    - Messages we receive from family, friends, teachers, religious leaders, stories, childhood experiences, TV, movies, books, and so on
- The Second Step
  - Identifying group membership
    - This occurs the moment two people meet
    - We live in a race conscious society and are conditioned to instinctively identify the group to which another person belongs
- The Third Step
  - Retrieving triggered stereotypes
    - Within milliseconds we retrieve the **most dominant associations** we have stored about that person's racial or ethnic group
    - These stereotypes are triggered and are used in shaping our understanding of the situation, regardless of the accuracy
- The Fourth Step
  - Activating implicit biases
    - Group stereotypes that have formed over time based upon our stored social knowledge

        - For example, thinking or saying a particular racially or ethnically diverse group is lazy
    - These unconscious stereotypes pulled out of storage judge the person or situation before us regardless of the accuracy or applicability to the person at hand
        - This is harmful as it is erroneous and devalues individual characteristics
        - This demonstrates the power of labeling and judging someone inaccurately
- The Fifth Step
    - Forming biased perceptions
        - Our stored stereotypes completely displace and supersede new or even contradictory information as we meet new people and encounter new situations
- The Sixth Step
    - Influencing
        - Implicit bases influence our perceptions, judgments, and actions and direct how we engage and interact

(Matthew, 2015)

Neuroscience of Implicit Bias

The amygdala is the region of the brain associated with emotions and fear (Kubota et al., 2012). It is the portion of the brain associated with the fight or flight response (Kubota et al., 2012). Research using functional magnetic resonance imaging has provided insight into how we respond to biases at a neural level, and how biases activate areas of our brain associated with threat and fear (Reihl et al., 2015). Stronger implicit pro-White bias, as measured by the IAT, results in greater activation in the amygdala when viewing a Black face than when looking at a White face, indicating that these implicit responses are mediated at least in part by the amygdala (Phelps et al., 2000).

The science of neuroplasticity is promising in that it has demonstrated that different short- and long-term experiences can change the brain's structure (Agarwal, 2020). Social attitudes and stereotypes can change how the brain processes information (Kubota et al., 2012). Moreover, internal goals and other stimuli in the environment can alter the neurocircuitry of race (Kubota et al., 2012).

Brain-based differences in behavioral characteristics and cognitive skills can change across time and place meaning that our unconscious biases are learned through experiences and can also be unlearned (Agarwal, 2020).

Essential Facts

Aversive Racism: Avoidance of a group because they make you feel uncomfortable and you can, therefore, maintain the stereotypes of the groups (Davido, 2015). Aversive racists have very low explicit bias scores and very high implicit bias scores (Matthew, 2015; Penner et al., 2010). They deny expressly racist views and disapprove of racism in others while harboring unconscious racial prejudice (Matthew, 2015; Penner et al., 2010).

ACTIONS TO ADDRESS IMPLICIT BIAS

Most healthcare providers are unaware of their implicit biases and their effects. Implicit bias does not show up as blatant racist attitudes and behaviors (Blair et al., 2011; Penner, 2014). Rather, implicit bias shows up in subtle verbal and nonverbal communications and behaviors that providers do not consciously control. It may look like discomfort with Black patients and not outright hostility (Blair et al., 2011; Penner, 2014).

Raising awareness is important. However, simply offering coursework is not enough. Individual-level approaches to combat bias, such as antibias education programs, have only limited impact (Wood, 2020). Further there must be strong, committed, and sustained institutional support (Penner et al., 2014; Wood, 2020). Even when there is an awareness of racial disparities in healthcare, providers may not recognize how implicit biases contribute to these disparities.

Recommendations:

- Treat patients and colleagues as individuals
  - See each person as a unique individual rather than mainly as a representative of a racial or social group
    - Focusing also on the individual characteristics of a Black person—as a unique human being—can reduce the activation of erroneous racial stereotypes that can unfairly lower the quality of care
  - Value their identity as the person they are
- Engage in person-centered communication
  - Develop positive interpersonal relationships
  - Acknowledge and respect the unique qualities of an individual
- Practice joint decision-making
  - The provider and the patient have shared power and responsibility

- Acknowledge and address uncomfortable feelings and thoughts
  - Do not suppress these feelings
  - Consider specific feelings, thoughts, and reactions to individuals or groups as potential indicators of implicit bias
  - Consider how these feelings, thoughts, and reactions might affect your actions and decisions

(Blair et al., 2011; IHI Multimedia Team, 2017)

CASE STUDY

Ebele is doing her final capstone rotation in a small community hospital. One of the patients is a 21-year-old Black male with splenic contusion and fractures of the left femur, tibia, and fibula status post an automobile accident. Ebele's preceptor tells her to be careful with those types of patients when giving pain medication because they probably have a history of substance use disorder. Ebele asked her preceptor to clarify what she meant by those types of patients. The preceptor said you know, young, Black male. They are all alike. Ebele then reminded the preceptor that they took the patient's history together earlier in the day and the patient denied a history of drug use.

Ebele then said this is a small community hospital where most of the patients are White. How many Black males do you see on this unit? The preceptor said he was the first young Black patient she had taken care of since being on the unit for over a year. Ebele tells the preceptor that as a Black woman she is offended by her comments. In addition, she tells her that her attitudes, language, and actions contribute to disparities in care for Black patients. Further Ebele explains how implicit bias leads to excess morbidity and mortality for Black patients.

Case Study Questions

1. The preceptor made a judgment based on a stereotype. How may societal stereotypes influence your attitudes and behaviors in clinical and learning environments?
2. Can you recall a recent situation in the learning or clinical environment where you were aware of your implicit biases?
3. How often do you have conversations about implicit bias where you work?

REFERENCES

Agarwal, P. (2020). What neuroimaging can tell us about our unconscious biases. *Scientific American*. Retrieved May 10, 2021, from https://blogs.scientificamerican.com/observations/what-neuroimaging-can-tell-us-about-our-unconscious-biases/

Blair, I. V., Steiner, J. F., & Havranek, E. P. (2011). Unconscious (implicit) bias and health disparities: Where do we go from here? *Permenente Journal, 15*(2), 71–78.

Chapman, E. N., Kaatz, A., & Carnes, M. (2013). Physicians and implicit bias: How doctors may unwittingly perpetuate health care disparities. *Journal of General Internal Medicine, 28*(11), 504–1510.

Davido, J. (2015). *Speaking of psychology: Understanding you racial biases.* American Psychological Association, Episode 31. Retrieved May 10, 2021, from https://www.apa.org/research/action/speaking-of-psychology/understanding-biases

FitzGerald, C., & Hurst, S. (2017). Implicit bias in health care professionals: A systematic review. *BMC Medical Ethics, 18*(1), 1–18. https://doi.org/10.1186/s12910-017-0179-8

Green, A. R., Carney, D. R., Pallin, D. J., Ngo, L. H., Raymond, K. L., Iezzoni, L. I., & Banaji, M. R. (2007). Implicit bias among physicians and its prediction of thrombolysis decisions for black and white patients. *Journal of General Internal Medicine, 22*(9), 1231–1238. https://doi.org/10.1007/s11606-007-0258-5

Greenwald, A. G., & Krieger, L. H. (2006). Implicit bias: Scientific foundations. *California Law Review, 94*(4), 945–968.

Greenwald, A. G., McGhee, D. E., & Schwartz, J. L. K. (1998). Measuring individual differences in implicit cognition: The implicit association test. *Journal of Personality and Social Psychology, 74*(6), 1464–1480.

Greenwald, A. G. & Banaji, M. R. (1995). Implicit social cognition: Attitudes, self-esteem, and stereotypes. *Psychological Review, 102*(1), 4–27.

Hall, W. J., Chaman, M. V., Lee, K. M., Merino, Y. M., Thomas, T. W., Payne, B. K., Eng, E., Day, S. H., & Coyne-Beasley, T. (2015). Implicit racial/ethnic bias among health care professionals and its influence on healthcare outcomes: A systematic review. *American Journal of Public Health, 105*(12), e60–e76.

IHI Multimedia Team. (2017, September 28). *How to reduce implicit bias.* Institute for Healthcare Improvement. http://www.ihi.org/communities/blogs/how-to-reduce-implicit-bias

Kirwan Institute. (2018). *Implicit bias module series.* Kirwan institute for the Study of Race and Ethnicity. Retrieved May 5, 2021, from http://kirwaninstitute.osu.edu/implicit-bias-training/

Kubota, J. T., Banaji, M. R., & Phelps, E. A. (2012). The neuroscience of race. *Nature Neuroscience, 15*(7), 940–948.

Mason, B. (2020, June 4). Curbing implicit bias: What works and what doesn't. *Knowable Magazine.* https://knowablemagazine.org/article/mind/2020/how-to-curb-implicit-bias

Matthew, D. B. (2015). *Just medicine: A cure for racial inequality in American Health Care.* NYU Press, JSTOR. Retrieved October 23, 2020, from www.jstor.org/stable/j.ctt15zc6c8

Morning Edition. (2016, October 17). *How the concept of implicit bias came into being.* NPR. https://www.npr.org/2016/10/17/498219482/how-the-concept-of-implicit-bias-came-into-being

Nosek, B. A., Banaji, M. R., & Greenwald, A. G. (2002). Harvesting implicit group attitudes and beliefs from a demonstration web site. *Group Dynamics: Theory, Research, and Practice*, *6*(1), 101–115. https://doi.org/10.1037/1089-2699.6.1.101

Penner, L. A., Dovidio, J. F., West, T. V., Gaertner, S. L., Albrecht, T. L., Dailey, R. K., & Markova, T. (2010). Aversive racism and medical interactions with Black patients: A field study. *Journal of Experimental Social Psychology*, *46*(2), 436–440.

Penner, L. A., Dovidio, J. F., Gonzalez, R., Albrecht, T. L., Chapman, R., Foster, T., Harper, F. W. K., Hagiwara, N., Hamel, L. M., Shields, A. F., Gadgeel, S., Simon, M. S., & Griggs, J. J. (2016). The effects of oncologist implicit racial bias in racially discordant oncology interactions. *Journal of Clinical Oncology*, *34*(24), 2874–2880. https://doi.org/10.1200/JCO.2015.66.3658

Phelps, E. A., O'Connor, K. J., Cunningham, W. A., Funayama, E. S., Gatenby, J. C., Gore, J. C., & Banaji, M. R. (2000). Performance on indirect measures of race evaluation predicts amygdala activation. *Journal of Cognitive Neuroscience*, *12*, 729–738.

Project Implicit. (2011). Frequently asked questions. Retrieved May, 2021, from https://implicit.harvard.edu/implicit/faqs.html

Reihl, K. M., Hurley, R. A., & Taber, K. H. (2015). Neurobiology of implicit and explicit bias: Implications for clinicians. *Journal of Neuropsychiatry and Clinical Neuroscience*, *27*(4), 248–253.

Schulman, K. A., Berlin, J. A., Harless, W., Kerner, J. F., Sistrunk, S., Gersh, B. J., Dube, R., Taleghani, C. K., Burke, J. E., Williams, S., Eisenberg, M. D., Ayers, W., & Escarce, J. J. (1999). The effect of race and sex on physicians recommendations for cardiac catheterization. *New England Journal of Medicine*, *340*, 618–626.

Scientific American Frontiers. (2015, April 2). The hidden prejudice. https://www.youtube.com/watch?v=3Nj-MjBc-xQ

Smedley, B. D., Stith, A. Y., & Nelson, A. R. (2003). *Unequal treatment: Confronting racial and ethnic disparities in health care.* The National Academies Press.

Whitehead, M., & Dahlgren, G. (2006). *Concepts and principles for tackling social inequities in health: Levelling up part 1.* University of Liverpool, WHO Collaborating Centre for Policy Research on Social Determinants of Health. www.who.int/social_determinants/resources/levelling_up_part1.pdf

Wood, J. L. (2020, February 4). When they say: "Implicit bias trainings don't work." *Diverse Issues in Higher Education*. https://www.diverseeducation.com/opinion/article/15106199/when-they-say-implicit-bias-trainings-dont-work

Ziegert, J. C., & Hanges, P. J. (2005). Employment discrimination: The role of implicit attitudes, motivation, and a climate for racial bias. *Journal of Applied Psychology*, *90*(3), 355–562.

10

Microaggressions

"It isn't about having your feelings hurt. It's about how being repeatedly dismissed and alienated and insulted and invalidated reinforces the differences in power and privilege, and how this perpetuates racism and discrimination."

—Roberto Montenegro

There was once a time when we made excuses for those who engaged in microaggressive behavior. We said things like "Oh, they didn't mean it," "You're being too sensitive," or "Get over it." The acceptance, silence, complicity, and passivity need to stop. Gone are those days when we did not challenge microaggressions because we believed they were harmless and insignificant. Given the immense physical, emotional, and psychological harm inflicted by these on-going occurrences rooted in racism and connected to implicit bias, bias, and discrimination we must all understand microaggressive behavior, know when we are engaging in it, and be vigilant to own, disrupt, dismantle, and disarm these destructive words and behaviors.

After reading this chapter, the reader will be able to:

1. Define the types of racial microaggressions
2. Explain the harmful effects of microaggressions
3. Discuss microinterventions for responding to microaggressions
4. Discuss accountability, responsibility, and owning microaggressive behavior

5. Discuss the importance of self-care when dealing with micro aggressions
6. Explain actions for disrupting microaggressive behavior
7. Examine the role of allies and bystanders in disarming micro aggressions

An internet search for the term *microaggression* generally results in a definition along the lines of: *a term used for brief everyday verbal or nonverbal slights, snubs, or insults that, whether intentional or unintentional, are directed toward an individual due to their group identity and communicate hostile, derogatory, or negative messages* (Sue et al., 2007). The definition is usually followed by a brief sentence that gives credit to the originator of the term: *Dr. Chester Pierce first coined the term in the 1970s to describe the subtle racial putdowns experienced by Black Americans* (Pierce et al., 1978).

Essential Facts

Solorzano et al. (2000) conducted one of the first empirical studies to examine racial microaggressions experienced by African Americans. The researchers used grounded theory for a qualitative study that explored the racial microaggressions and campus climate for 34 African American students who attended three elite, predominately White, Research I Universities in the United States. Themes that emerged from the focus groups were invisibility in the classroom, lowered educational expectations by faculty, and racial segregation. The participants also reported experiencing racial microaggressions outside of the classroom and unspoken double standards.

While generally understood that (a) microaggressions are directed toward an individual or group due to culturally marginalized identities such as gender identity, sexual orientation, race, class, or immigration status, and that (b) Chester Pierce first coined the term, the significance of the concept cannot be fully comprehended without elucidation of the original intent of the term and knowledge of the life of the man who first introduced the concept.

CHESTER PIERCE

Chester Pierce graduated from Harvard Medical School in 1952. His goal was to achieve excellence in every way possible (West, 1983). Dr. Pierce was a physician, psychiatrist, researcher, and an academician (West, 1983). Much of Dr. Pierce's work focused on things that he experienced and understood such as extreme environments, racism, and resilience (Bell, 1998). Pierce described microaggressions as "subtle, stunning, often automatic, and non-verbal exchanges which are 'put downs' of Blacks by offenders" (Pierce et al., 1978, p. 66).

DERALD WING SUE

Derald Wing Sue did much of the pioneering work on racial microaggressions (Sue et al., 2007). He developed a framework for conceptualizing microaggressions that is grounded in a combination of empirical and experimental research, professional literature, and personal narratives (Sue et al., 2007).

Sue defines racial microaggressions as the brief and everyday slights, insults, indignities and denigrating messages sent to people of color by well-intentioned White people who are unaware of the hidden messages being communicated (Sue et al., 2007).

It is important to note that microaggressions occur not only as interpersonal human interactions, but they are also environmental in nature (Sue et al., 2007). A human or interpersonal microaggression is asking an Asian individual multiple times where they are from and not accepting their first response of "the United States" (Sue et al., 2007). Environmental macroaggressions involve the exclusion of underrepresented groups from the public arena and from things such as books, statues, movies, advertising, accepted standards of beauty, and the naming of buildings (Sue et al., 2007).

RACIAL MICROAGGRESSIONS

Sue et al., 2007 describes racial microaggressions as reflections of the world views of inclusion, exclusion, superiority, inferiority, that come out in ways that are outside the level of conscious awareness of an individual.

Racial microaggressions are different from everyday rudeness in that they are:

- Constant and continual in the lives of people of color
- Cumulative in nature and represent a lifelong burden of stress
- Continuous reminders of their second-class status in society
- Symbolic of past governmental injustices directed toward people of color, such as the enslavement of Black people, incarceration of Japanese Americans, and appropriating land from Native Americans (Sue et al., 2007)

Sue describes three forms of racial macroaggressions.

Microassults are conscious, explicit, discriminatory actions that are purposeful and meant to hurt the intended person. They have been referred to as old fashioned racism that's done on a one-on-one level. The behaviors may range from derogatory name calling to avoidant behavior (Sue et al., 2007).

Thoughts of minority inferiority are usually private. Therefore, microassults usually happen in private where the person engaged in the microaggressive behavior can remain anonymous. It is believed that when microassults are publicly displayed the person exhibiting microaggressive behavior has lost control or feels safe in an environment to engage in microassults (Sue et al., 2007).

Microinsults are unconscious acts. They are rude and insensitive and demean a person's racial heritage or identity. While microinsults clearly deliver an insulting hidden message to the recipient of color, these subtle snubs are generally unknown to the person delivering the microinsult. Two commonly experienced examples are when a White person on a search committee says, *I believe the most qualified person should get the job, regardless of race or when an employee of color is asked, How did you land this job?* The underlying message from the perspective of a person of color is (a) people of color are not believed to be qualified and (b) you must have gotten the position because of some type of affirmative action or quota program, not because of your ability. Hearing these statements frequently makes the recipient likely to experience such statements as microaggressions (Sue et al., 2007).

Microinsults may also be nonverbal and may convey to individuals of color that their contributions are not important. Examples are when a White professor tends not to acknowledge students of color in the classroom or appears nervous, distracted, and avoids eye contact when speaking with students of color (Sue et al., 2007).

Microinvalidations are the most common type of racial microaggression (Table 10.1). They are subtle and characterized by the exclusion, negation, or the nullification of thoughts, feelings, and lived experiences of a person of color (Figure 10.1). Common examples include (a) Asian Americans, born and raised in the United States being complimented for "speaking really good English" or repeatedly asking where they were born, which negates their U.S. American heritage and makes them feel like foreigners in their own land. (b) Black people being told "I don't see color" or "We are all human beings." These expressions negate their experiences as Black people. (c) When a LatinX couple receives poor service at a restaurant and shares the experience with friends only to be told, "You are just being too sensitive." The couple is being nullified and the reality of their experience is being nullified (Sue et al., 2007).

Table 10.1

Examples of Racial Microaggressions

Theme	Microaggression	Message
Alien in own land When Asian Americans and Latino Americans are assumed to be foreign born	"Where are you from?" "Where were you born?" "You speak good English." A person asking an Asian American to teach them words in their native language	You are not American. You are a foreigner.
Ascription of intelligence Assigning intelligence to a person of color on the basis of their race	"You are a credit to your race." "You are so articulate." Asking an Asian person to help with a math or science problem	People of color are generally not as intelligent as Whites. It is unusual for someone of your race to be intelligent. All Asians are intelligent and good in math/sciences.
Color blindness Statements that indicate that a White person does not want to acknowledge race	"When I look at you, I don't see color." "America is a melting pot." "There is only one race, the human race."	Denying a person of color's racial/ethnic experiences Assimilate/acculturate to the dominant culture Denying the individual as a racial/cultural being
Criminality/assumption of criminal status	A White man or woman clutching their purse or checking their wallet as a Black or Latino approaches or passes A store owner following a customer of color around the store A White person waits to ride the next elevator when a person of color is on it.	You are a criminal. You are going to steal/you are poor/you do not belong. You are dangerous.
Denial of individual racism A statement made when Whites deny their racial biases	"I'm not racist. I have several Black friends." "As a woman, I know what you go through as a racial minority."	I am immune to racism because I have friends of color. Your racial oppression Is no different than my gender oppression. I can't be a racist. I'm like you.

(continued)

Table 10.1

Examples of Racial Microaggressions (*continued*)

Theme	Microaggression	Message
Myth of meritocracy Statements which assert that race does not play a role in life successes	"I believe the most qualified person should get the job.' "Everyone can succeed in this society, if they work hard enough."	People of color are given extra unfair benefits because of their race. People of color are lazy and/or incompetent and need to work harder.
Pathologizing cultural values/ communication styles The notion that the values and communication styles of the dominant/White culture are ideal	Asking a Black person: "Why do you have to be so loud/ animated? Just calm down." To an Asian or Latino person: "Why are you so quiet? We want to know what you think. Be more verbal." "Speak up more.' Dismissing an individual who brings up race/culture in a work/school setting	Assimilate to dominant culture Leave your cultural baggage outside.
Second-class citizen Occurs when a White person is given preferential treatment as a consumer over a person of color	Person of color mistaken for a service worker Having a taxi cab pass a person of color and pick up a White passenger Being ignored at a store counter as attention is given to the White customer behind you "You people…"	People of color are servants to Whites. They couldn't possibly occupy high-status positions. You are likely to cause trouble and/or travel to a dangerous neighborhood. Whites are more valued customers than people of color. You don't belong. You are a lesser being.
Environmental microaggressions Macro-level microaggressions, which are more apparent on systemic and environmental levels	A college or university with buildings that are all named after White, heterosexual, upper class males. Television shows and movies that feature predominantly White people, without representation of people of color Overcrowding of public schools in communities of color Overabundance of liquor stores in communities of color	You don't belong/you won't succeed here. There is only so far you can go. You are an outsider/you don't exist. People of color don't/ shouldn't value education. People of color are deviant.

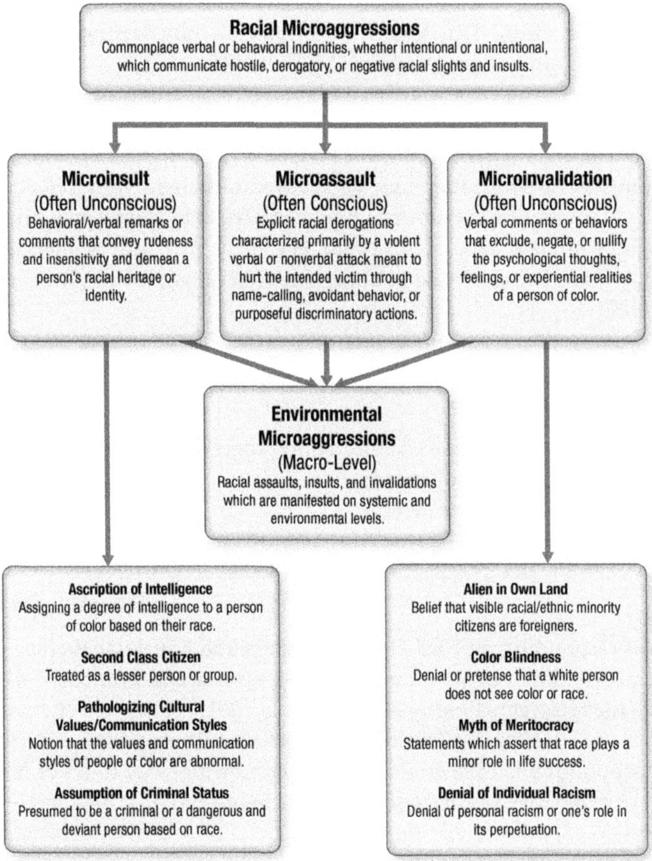

Figure 10.1 Categories of and Relationships Among Racial Microaggressions.

The Harmful Impact of Microaggressions

The harmful health effects of microaggressions cannot be understated (Nadal, 2014; Sue et al., 2007, 2019). The full magnitude of their destructive nature must be fully elucidated and comprehended. Moreover, their harmful impact must not be downplayed. Microinsults and microinvalidations put people of color in a psychological bind that is painful, isolating, and exhausting (Sue, 2010).

When a person of color confronts someone who has directed a microaggression toward them, the deliverer of the microaggression will usually deny it (Sue, 2010). In fact, the person who delivered the microaggression usually does not acknowledge that anything has happened because they are not aware that they are being offensive (Sue, 2010). This leaves the person of color feeling insulted, confused, and angry (Nadal, 2014; Sue, 2010).

Responding with anger to a microaggression and striking back may be a healthy reaction. However, it may result in negative consequences for a person of color (Sue et al., 2008). When persons of color do respond, they may be accused of being overly sensitive, or their emotional outbursts may confirm held stereotypes about people of color (Sue et al., 2008). For Black men and women this may mean being labeled as angry, aggressive, or violent (Sue et al., 2008).

Conversely, a person of color may decide to do nothing and hold their anger inside. This response occurs because a person of color may be:

- Unable to determine whether a microaggression has occurred
- At a loss for how to respond
- Fearful of the consequences
- Rationalizing that "it won't do any good anyway"
- Engaging in self-deception through denial: It didn't happen

(Sue et al., 2019)

Not responding may lead to helplessness and hopelessness (Sue et al., 2019). Microaggressions can cause a *freeze effect* for those who are the recipients (Sousa, 2018; Sue et al., 2019). This lack of action may lead to later rumination and negative self-evaluation and self-disappointment (Sue et al., 2019). Not knowing what to do or how to respond may cause those on the receiving end of a microaggression to experience extreme guilt, anxiety, or self-disappointment (Sue et al., 2019). Moreover, doing nothing denies one's lived reality and it erodes one's integrity and the pent-up anger and frustration takes its toll psychologically and physically and emotionally (Sue et al., 2019).

Overall, the harmful impact of microaggressions include:

- Lower self-esteem
- Increased anger and frustration
- Decreased mental and physical energy
- Increased risk of health problems
- Shortened life expectancy
- Denied equal access to opportunity (including but not limited to education, employment, and healthcare)
- Feelings of difference
- Internalized stigma
- Fear of rejection

- Lower utilization and premature termination of services (psychological or otherwise)
- Increased stress
- Mistrust within a community
- Lack of safety

(Sue et al., 2019)

Responding to Microaggressions

While we need for people not to engage in microaggressive behavior, it happens (Carter & McMillian-Bohler, 2021). Therefore, until microaggressions become less of an accepted way of being in our society, we must have strategies for how to respond to them (Carter & McMillian-Bohler, 2021). Deciding whether or not to respond to a microaggression and then knowing what to say or how to behave can be taxing (Sue et al., 2019).

Sue created a list of responses to microaggressions that include:

- Passivity, retreat, or give up
- Strike back or hurt the aggressor
- Stop, diminish, deflect, or put an end to the harmful act
- Educate the perpetrator
- Validate and support people on the receiving end
- Act as an ally
- Seek social support
- Enlist outside authority or institutional intervention
- Any combination of the above

(Sue et al., 2019)

Sue further organized the responses into strategic goals for responding to microaggressions:

- To make the invisible visible
- To disarm the microaggression
- To educate the perpetrator
- To seek external reinforcement or support

(Sue et al., 2019)

Microinterventions are words or deeds, whether intentional or unintentional, that communicate to the recipient of microaggressions (a) validation of their experiential reality, (b) value as a person, (c) affirmation of their racial or group identity, (d) support and encouragement, and (e) reassurance that they are not alone. Microinterventions are interpersonal tools that can be used to disarm or counteract the effects of microaggressions by challenging and educating those who deliver them (Sue et al., 2019).

Recipients of Microaggressions

Because microaggressions happen so quickly, it is important to be prepared with counteracting responses (Nadal, 2014). The decision to respond to a microaggression is a personal decision. Questions to ask when deciding whether or not to respond include:

- If I respond, could my physical safety be in danger?
- If I respond, will the person become defensive and will this lead to an argument?
- If I respond, how will this affect my relationship with this person (e.g., coworker, family member)?
- Will responding affect my job or school status if I respond?
- If I don't respond, will I regret not saying something?
- If I don't respond, does that convey that I accept the behavior or statement?

(Nadal, 2014)

Researchers have developed several approaches for managing microaggressions.

The **O**pen **T**he **F**ront **D**oor to Communication is a microresistance framework that has four steps:

- **O**bserve: Concrete, factual, and observable
  - State what you observed in very concrete and factual manner
    - "I noticed…"
- Think:
  - Express your thoughts based on observation
    - "I think…"
  - Feel:
    - State your emotions,
      - "I feel…"
- Desire:
  - Make a specific request or inquire about desired outcome
    - "I would like…

(Harvard Macy Institute, 2019)

Another strategy involves memorizing three prepared statements.

- **Ask for more clarification:**
  - "Could you say more about what you mean by that?" "How have you come to think that?"
- **Separate intent from impact:**
  - "I know you didn't realize this, but when you __________ (comment/behavior), it was hurtful/offensive because___________. Instead you could___________ (suggest different language or behavior)."

- **For Allies: Share your own process:**
  - "I noticed that you ___________ (comment/behavior). I used to do/say that too, but then I learned_____________."

(Yoon, 2020)

Deliverers of Microaggressions

There needs to be increased awareness and sensitivity of all people to microaggressions so that they accept responsibility for their behaviors and for changing them (Nadal, 2014; Sue et al., 2019). When a person delivers a microaggression and the recipient or an ally or a bystander confronts the communication or behavior, it is important for the deliverer to listen without becoming defensive (Nadal, 2014; Sue et al., 2019). The worst thing is to deny that the recipient is hurt or offended. Invalidating their experience is a microaggression in itself (Nadal, 2014). Think about what was said and how it made the recipient feel based upon the feedback that is being given (Nadal, 2014). Reflect on how what was said could have been delivered in a more positive way (Nadal, 2014). Moreover, own up to it (Nadal, 2014). Admit that a microaggression was committed, learn from the wrongdoing, and genuinely apologize (Nadal, 2014).

- Learn constant vigilance of your own biases and fears
- Experiential reality is important in interacting with people who are different from you in terms of race, culture, and ethnicity
- Don't be defensive
- Be open to discussing your own attitudes and biases and how they might have hurt others or in some sense might reveal bias on your part
- Be an ally: Stand personally against all forms of bias and discrimination

(Sue, 2010)

Allies are individuals who belong to dominant social groups and, through their support of nondominant groups, actively work toward the eradication of prejudicial practices they witness in both their personal and professional lives (Sue et al., 2019). Allies are more likely to have an awareness of themselves as racial beings that has evolved over time and generally have some understanding of the sociopolitical construction of race and racism.

Bystanders are anyone who witness microaggressions that are worthy of comment or action. Bystanders generally do not recognize bias and discrimination as racism and lack an awareness of institutional racism and how it operates. Inaction and passivity are generally the norm for bystanders.

Take Care of Yourself

Constant racial microaggressions in the lived experiences of people of color have been described as a chronic state of Racial Battle Fatigue (Sue et al., 2019). Emotion-focused (internal self-care) and problem-focused (external, cause of the stress) coping strategies for dealing with chronic stress have been elucidated in the literature (Lazarus & Folkman, 1984).

Supportive communication about microaggressions facilitates self-care. Discussing common experiences with friends or in a more structured environment such as a support group is recommended.

Context matters; always consider your safety and consider the context and the environmental conditions. Moreover, ask if there are specific instances when interventions would be harmful by reducing self-efficacy and autonomy or by increasing microaggressions?

Microintervention Cautions

- *Pick your battles.*
  - Responding to frequent microaggressions can be exhausting and energy depleting.
  - For self-preservation and safety, determine which offense or abuse is worthy of action and effort.
- *Consider where and when you choose to address the offender.*
  - Calling someone out in public may provoke defensiveness or cause a situation that increases the microaggressions.
  - Determine the place (public or private) and time (immediate or later) to respond.
- *Adjust your response as the situation warrants.*
  - If something was said or done out of ignorance, *educate* rather than just *confront.*
- *Be aware of relationship factors and dynamics.*
  - Interventions may vary depending on the relationship to the aggressor. Is the culprit a family member, friend, coworker, stranger, or superior? Each relationship may dictate a different response. For a close family member, education may have a higher priority than for a stranger.
- *Always consider the consequences of microinterventions, especially when a strong power differential exists between the deliverer and the recipient.*
  - Although positive results can ensue from a microintervention, there is always the potential for negative outcomes that place the recipient, ally, or bystander at risk.

(Sue et al., 2019)

CASE STUDY

Mikala started her new position as a nurse practitioner (NP) on the critical care unit of a large teaching hospital with excitement and enthusiasm. She had always worked in small community settings and, after completing a DNP program, relocated across the country for this new opportunity. Mikala graduated at the top of her class. She was outspoken, friendly, and thrived in high-paced, high-acuity environments. She quickly became lead NP on the service. Mikala noticed, however, that when rounding with the interprofessional team the attending physician never looks her directly in the eye when she is speaking. The attending does not acknowledge her contributions and dismisses her questions. The attending's attitude and behavior toward her makes others on the team uncomfortable, however, no one says anything. Makala spends her hour drive home in the evenings wondering what she should do about the situation. She knows it cannot continue and that she must address the behavior. As the only Black person on the team, she feels marginalized, devalued, and invisible. She is annoyed that so much of her time and mental energy is now spent on this situation.

Case Study Questions

1. As a colleague what would be your role as an **ally** in promoting equity and dismantling racism?
2. What are Mikala's options for addressing this situation?
3. What health risks are being exhibited by Mikala due to exposure to racial microaggressions?

REFERENCES

Bell, C. C. (1998). Race, psychiatry. *Journal of the American Medical Association*, *280*(8), 752–723.

Carter, B., & McMillian-Bohler, J. (2021). Rewriting the microaggression narrative: Enhancing nursing students' ability to respond. *Nurse Educator*, *46*(2), 6–100.

Harvard Macy Institute. (2019, May 20). Microresistance. https://www.harvardmacy.org/index.php/hmi/microresistance

Lazarus, R. S., & Folkman, S. (1984). *Stress, appraisal, and coping.* Springer Publishing Company.

Nadal, K. L. 2014. A guide to responding to microaggressio'n's. *CUNY Forum*, *2*(1), 71–76.

Pierce, C., Carew, J., Pierce-Gonzalez, D., & Wills, D. (1978). An experiment in racism: TV commercials. *Education and Urban Society, 10*(1), 61–87.

Solorzano, D., Ceja, M., & Yosso, T. (2000). Critical race theory, racial microaggressions, and campus racial climate: The experiences of African American college students. *Journal of Negro Education, 69*, 60–73.

Sousa, T. (2018, April 30). *Responding to microaggressions in the classroom.* Magna Publications. https://www.facultyfocus.com/articles/effective-classroom-management/responding-to-microaggressions-in-the-classroom/

Sue, D. W., Alsaidi, S., Awad, M. N., Glaeser, E., Calle, C. Z., & Mendez, N. (2019). Disarming racial microaggressions: Microintervention strategies for targets, white allies, and bystanders. *American Psycholigst, 74*(1), 128–142.

Sue, D. W. (2010). *Microaggressions in everyday life: Race, gender & sexual orientation*. Wiley.

Sue, D. W., Capodilupo, C. M., Torino, G. C., Bucceri, J. M., Holder, A. M. B., Nadal, K. L., & Esquilin, M. (2007). Racial microaggressions in everyday life: Implications for clinical practice. *American Psychologist, 62*, 271–286. http://dx.doi.org/10.1037/0003-066X.62.4.271

Sue, D. W., Nadal, K. L., Capodiluop, C. M., Lin, A. I., Torino, G. C., & Rivera, D. P. (2008). Racial microaggressions against Black Americans: Implications for counseling. *Journal of Counseling & Development, 86*, 330–338.

West, L. J. (1983). Chester Middlebrook Pierce, M.D., Sc.D. *American Journal of Orthopsychiatry, 53*(2), 196–200.

Yoon, H. (2020, March 3). How to respond to microaggressions. *The New York Times.* https://www.nytimes.com/2020/03/03/smarter-living/how-to-respond-to-microaggressions.html

11

Becoming the "Nurse-Citizen"

"Activism is my rent for living on this planet."

—Alice Walker (n.d.)

In 1972, James Baldwin, cautioned that, "ignorance, allied with power, is the most ferocious enemy justice can have" (p. 445). Fifty years later, clinicians are recognizing this moment of reckoning and addressing our country's structural and systemic racism. Nurses have both an opportunity and a responsibility to look beyond our institutional walls and the healthcare system and actively engage with our fellow citizens in creating a just and equitable society for all. It is now widely recognized that "racism is a public health crisis" (Acosta, 2020; American Nurses Association [ANA], 2020; Yearby, 2020), so if nurses (as members of the most trusted profession in America) are truly committed to addressing social and structural determinants of health, we must advocate not only for more effective health policy, but improvements to all public policy.

After reading this chapter, the reader will be able to:

1. Explain the history of the definition of a nurse-citizen
2. Discuss the history of select nurse-citizens and their impact on organizations, communities, and policy
3. Reflect on examples of nurse-citizens who took action during the extraordinary 2020 Year of the Nurse
4. Discuss ways in which each of us can become nurse-citizens and work to promote inclusive excellence and racial equity

DEFINITIONS OF THE NURSE-CITIZEN OVER THE LAST 70 YEARS

- 1949: Faulkner called on all nurses to recognize their civic duty to create a society that guarantees equity for all and specifically called on nurses with their "enlightened conscience" to ensure that no patient be seen as "inferior" or experience discrimination (p. 26). Jones (1949) similarly argued that nurses, with their clinical training and focus on health promotion and care of the whole person, bring a unique perspective to community planning and budgeting and encouraged nurses to join her in the important role of nurse-citizen: "Given a natural interest in individuals, combined with experience as a nurse, plus pep and enthusiasm, a civic-minded woman can make a unique contribution to community life" (p. 616).
- 1989: Bevis noted, "The individual nurse-citizen has some control over and responsibility for the political and social milieu in which she lives" (p. 44).
- 2016: Manton described the importance of the *nurse-citizen* to engage in social and political action by:
    - Critically reviewing candidates and ballot measures and voting in every election
    - Speaking up in public meetings and/or committees and sharing our expert knowledge of the healthcare system and/or concerns we have about unmet health needs in the community
    - Joining with other nurses in political action through our professional organizations
- 2017: Clark and colleagues envisioned the *nurse-citizen* as one who is engaging in a "praxis embedded in meaningful work with just solutions, [and] enhancing the agency of all involved in promoting health and well-being" (p. 247).

HISTORY OF THE NURSE-CITIZEN

Our nursing profession has a long history of advocacy for social change (Mason et al., 2020). While many nursing schools cover Florence Nightingale and Lillian Wald and their civic work, few of us were taught about America's Black nurses who had looked beyond their individual practice to create long-lasting change in their communities and in the profession. More impressively, these nurses did so under the challenges of racism. Table 11.1 assembles a list of notable nurse-citizens and their inspiring accomplishments.

Table 11.1

Notable Nurse-Citizens

Nurse-Citizen	Inspiring Accomplishments
Florence Nightingale (National Trust, n.d.)	• Brought student nurses to care for the sick in the workhouse infirmaries where previously there had been able-bodied inmates to do the work • She used her social influence and statistics to lobby the government's *Poor Law Board* to improve the delivery of care to those in workhouses
Mary Elizabeth Mahoney (Wisconsin Center for Nursing, n.d.)	• First African American woman to graduate from nursing school • Cofounded the National Association of Colored Graduate Nurses (NACGN) and fought to end discrimination within the nursing profession • One of the first women in Boston to register to vote • American Nurses Association now has a biennial award in her name to honor those who work to advance equity among nurses
Mabel Keaton Staupers, RN (Staten, 2011)	• Fought to integrate Black nurses into the Army Nurse Corps during World War II • Lobbied (successfully) to fully integrate the American Nurses Association
Marie Branch, RN, NP (Gatrall, 2020)	• Co-directed the Free Clinic in Los Angeles (in allyship with her White male physician partner) • Developed the philosophy of "ethnic humanism" to promote inclusion, shared decision-making, and accountability to Black, Indigenous, and People of Color (BIPOC) communities • Considered to be "way ahead of her time" as she fought to improve nursing curricular content to more effectively support students and communities of color and co-wrote the book, *Providing Safe Nursing Care for Ethnic People of Color* with Phyllis Perry Paxton
General Hazel Johnson-Brown, PhD, RN (Langer, 2011)	• Was originally denied entrance into nursing school because of her race • First African American woman to become General and to command the Army Nurse Corps • Director of the Center for Health Policy at George Mason University • Head of the ANA's governmental relations unit; • "She was not a 'quiet dissenter'..."
Beverly Malone, PhD, RN, FAAN (NLN, 2022)	• National League for Nursing President and CEO • Two term president of the American Nurses Association • Deputy Assistant Secretary for Health within the U.S. Department of Health and Human Services • First African American General Secretary of the Royal College of Nursing in the UK • Frequently offers "her expert perspective and public testimony" to policymakers and congressional leaders

(continued)

Table 11.1

Nurse-Citizen Inspiring Accomplishments (*continued*)

Nurse-Citizen	Inspiring Accomplishments
Ernest Grant, PhD, RN, FAAN (Brusie, 2021)	• First male nurse to lead the American Nurses Association (ANA) • Led ANA (2020) in proclaiming racism as public health crisis • Consciously volunteered for a COVID-19 vaccine study to provide data on Black Americans and be a role model • Encouraged all nurses to engage in politics and advocacy

Essential Facts

When we focus on not only our own individual biases, but also take a critical approach to the social ecology of racism and bias in America, the shift from "person-blaming" can lead to the recognition that while there are longstanding structural barriers to health equity, we are all part of a system that needs to change. We commit to being part of the solution by joining our health professions colleagues and scientists in becoming clinician-citizens.

2020 THE YEAR OF THE NURSE: AN EXTRAORDINARY YEAR OF NURSES THAT LED CHANGE IN THEIR COMMUNITIES, STATES, AND THE NATION

In 2020, nursing celebrated Florence Nightingale's birthday bicentennial. And what a year it was for nurses, with COVID-19 challenging us and other healthcare professionals more than at any other time since the flu pandemic of 1918–1919. In addition to our fellow nurses and their inspiring work in hospitals across the United States, there were several other nurses who made national news for their work as nurse-citizens:

- Sheila McMillan, RN, was featured on the cover of *Time* Magazine (2020) to represent the many healthcare professionals who were named "Guardians of the Year" for their heroic work during the COVID-19 pandemic. In addition to providing health education to the school staff, students, and parents, and providing emergency nursing care, Ms. McMillan also collaborated with the Black Doctors COVID-19 Consortium to provide testing in the Black communities who were hardest hit (Hill, 2020).
- Congressional Representative Lauren Underwood, MSN, MPH, is not only the youngest woman elected to the House of Representatives, but co-chairs the Black Maternal Health

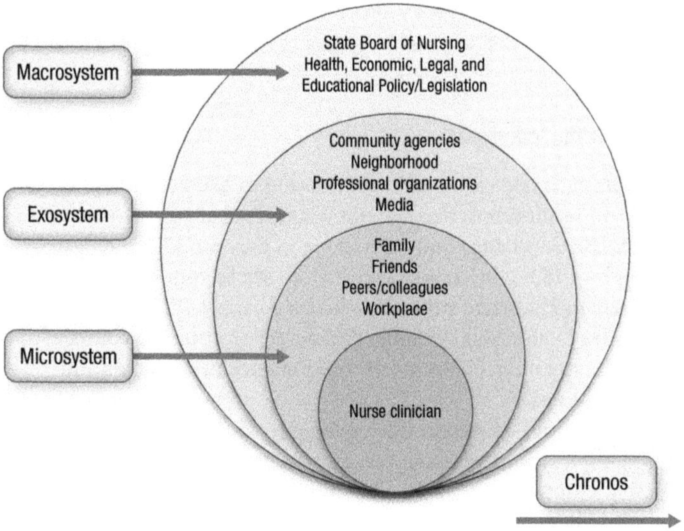

Figure 11.1 Brofenbrenner's (1977) Social Ecological Framework.

Caucus with Representative Alma Adams. She led the 2021 Momnibus legislation to address Black maternal health disparities and improve access to care and resources for all women (Momnibus, n.d.).

- Cori Bush, RN, grew up Missouri and, while used to seeing police abuse, she nevertheless became inspired to act after the murder of Michael Brown. She went on to become a leader of the Black Lives Matter movement, and was just recently the first Missouri nurse and first Black woman elected to the U.S. House of Representatives (Hardy, 2020).

Now let's revisit Brofenbrenner's Social Ecological Framework (1977) to imagine how and where we can join our fellow nurse-citizens in enacting sustainable change across the four systems (individual, micro, exo, and macro; Figure 11.1).

INDIVIDUAL

While our work to end population health disparities and systemic racism is critical to our role as a nurse-citizen, we cannot forget our role in the caring for the individual affected by these issues. Trappist Monk Thomas Merton (1969) offers sage advice for clinicians in addressing social and structural determinants of health: "If you want to identify me, ask me not where I live or what I like to eat, … ask me what I think is keeping me from living fully for the thing I want to live for" (p. 160).

Steps for the Individual

- Start each day with a daily affirmation or self-reflection. Take 5 to 10 minutes to think about Ghandi's challenge to each of us: "Be the change you wish to see in the world" and reflect on how to be the change you wish to see in your practice. Perhaps challenge yourself to be the formal and/or informal leader by thinking, valuing, and demonstrating the courage, understanding, compassion, and patience to all clients and communities.
- Be reflective-in-action during the day with this goal in mind. For example, take a moment before meeting with a client to consider the "chronos" of their life that has led them to seeking your care. At the end of the day, set aside time to reflect-on-action (e.g., by journaling, painting, talking with a mentor) about how you did. Just as we do in the nursing process when we evaluate our clients' goals, you can do the same and reflect on whether you achieved your goals. Part of the reflection process includes identifying the barriers and facilitators to those goals. Collecting these reflections over time will help more easily identify those factors that support or inhibit our efforts for building an antiracism practice.
- Finally, never give up and remember the sage words of Mary Church Terrell (NAACP founder and Black suffragist): "Lifting as we climb, onward and upward…" (Gailani, 2020) and to always help those around us to have the same opportunities to learn, grow, and achieve.

MICROSYSTEM

As we work on our own practice, remember that we have ecosystems that also impact our practice. Therefore, each of us should commit to trying our best each day to reach out to our colleagues and work collectively to identify the barriers and facilitators to creating health equity in our practice settings. Working in concert will help each of us be more strategic in our efforts and hopefully reduce potential "exercises in futility." Opportunities to connect with our colleagues include starting the day with an inspiring song or poem that celebrates both diversity and inclusiveness, working to increase our collective knowledge and understanding with journal/book/movie clubs, or developing more formalized monthly inclusion councils that work with the institution to promote sustainable change.

Essential Facts

We know that 80% of health is determined by factors outside clinical care. Armed with this knowledge and our ethical duty to advocate, all nurses must begin to look beyond their practice and institutional settings and toward more meaningful partnerships with community-based organizations and community members. The Prevention Institute (n.d.) has some excellent initiatives and resources.

For White nurses who are ready to ally with their Black, Indigenous, and People of Color (BIPOC) colleagues in creating change, but who might be afraid of saying or doing the wrong thing, Alicia Garza (2020) cautions against giving into fear, "Often people get deterred because they don't want to make mistakes. They don't want to say the wrong thing, and that keeps them from doing anything at all."

Some helpful ground rules for groups to consider include:

- Recognize and counter the divisiveness by looking at what unites us and to come together as Americans (see One America Guide [Franklin, & The Advisory Board to the President's Initiative on Race, 1998] in Chapter 12: Antiracism Multimedia Toolkit).
- Rely on a "calling in" versus "calling out" approach (Seed The Way, n.d.).
- Foster a "brave" learning space by willing to be vulnerable and embrace "controversy with civility" (Arao & Clemens, 2013, p. 144).

Other opportunities to be an institutional citizen could include:

- Work with your institution's quality improvement and/or patient outcomes committee to examine "health disparity" data such as preventable patterns of below-the-knee amputation rates, heart failure readmissions, super-utilizer cases, or hot spot zip codes. Next, develop a working group to engage in evidence-based practice projects for reducing these disparities.
- Partnering with your human resources colleagues to develop action plans for promoting inclusive excellence. The Office of the Governor of the Commonwealth of Virginia (2021) has an excellent "Strategic Plan for Inclusive Excellence" powerpoint that

includes a step-by-step process for organizations to develop output and outcome metrics for their diversity, equity, and inclusion programs.

Specific Strategies for Nurse Educators in Higher Education

For nurse educators in prelicensure, nurse residency, and graduate programs:

- Each generation of clinicians learns from the prior generation. If our generation and the ones before us never addressed the issue, how do we teach the next generation?
    - Work with your Office of Diversity, Equity, and Inclusion to organize "lunch and learn" forums for coming together and getting comfortable with the uncomfortable. Having experienced facilitators to guide the faculty's work is critical as students note that when such forums are not well-facilitated, they can cause more harm, "it's triggering and horrible, and people have really bad feelings" (Gonzalez et al., 2019, p. 696).
- The courage to speak up and call out "othering": We often hear in clinical practice and in class the "othering" of clients with stereotypes; for example, the frequent fliers, "those people," "inner-city," "tough clients," "drug-seeking". Teach students through role play or simulation the skills for calling-in versus calling-out. Seed The Way (n.d.) has easy to use documents for interrupting bias that educators can use to teach colleagues and students how to respond to bias and microaggressions.
- Understand microaggressions and their negative impact not only on clients but also on colleagues, whether it's feeling like you don't belong and/or experiencing "imposter syndrome" (Stone et al., 2018). McNair et al.'s (2020) *From Equity Talk to Equity Walk* provides faculty in higher education with a road map for creating a campus that fosters inclusive excellence and produces "equitable outcomes."
- Mitchell (2008) argues that we need to re-imagine Traditional Service-Learning with Critical Service-Learning (CSL). CSL uses a "critical approach" to service, encouraging students to question/examine existing power structures and hierarchies and to engage with the community in creating sustainable social change. Similarly, we could reimagine CSL by utilizing a critical social justice framework as proposed by Grain and Lund (2017) where students move from the traditional "charity" framework and toward one where they are embrace the "tension, ambiguity, and discomfort" as they work toward a conceptual space of "critical hope."

- Develop community-based learning courses in universities or continuing education series on health, society, and power where students can engage with community members and critically examine why there are still so many food deserts in our urban centers. Students and community members could also learn together about the emerging science of the microbiome, the importance of affordable nutrient-dense foods, and why food literacy and food policy are critical to health equity initiatives.

EXOSYSTEM

- Hakima Payne, MSN, RN, a labor and delivery nurse who witnessed racism at her institution, said "Black families were always held to a different standard, seen as more suspect. White patients were given leeway that Black patients were never given" (Krisberg, 2019). Her passion to see better care for Black families led her to create a more equitable and inclusive model of care for all: the Uzazi Village. Her "signature program," the Sister Doulas program, has successfully trained more than 100 doulas to provide comprehensive birthing support and postpregnancy care (Krisberg, 2019).
- Encouraging our institutions to partner with community-level organizations to optimize individual and community level equity. Virginia's Fairfax County Government (n.d.) provides an excellent practice guide for bringing together local stakeholders to create "opportunity neighborhoods." Butler et al. (2015) also provide an instructive case study on how health systems can collaboratively work with local partners to develop new models of data sharing, telehealth services, and case management programs that are cost-effective and improve the health of their communities. Nurses and their colleagues can use the Chronic Care Model as a framework for developing similar partnerships.
- Clinical researchers can utilize a community-based participatory approach when developing interventions designed to improve health equity. For example, look at the academic-community partnership the Wisconsin School of Nursing established: The Community Advisors on Research Design and Strategies (CARDS) program. In their model, the researchers are the learners and the community members are the teachers (Thomas et al., 2017).
- Clinical educators can work with the Association of Standardized Patient Educators (ASPE) and *Laerdal Medical* to revise their simulation cases so they allow the time and attention needed for students to go beyond the traditional "social history" (meso level)

of their family social supports and clue the student learner to consider the importance of public policy that impacts our clients' abilities to effectively manage their health and well-being.

- The most current Core Competencies for Interprofessional Education Collaborative (2016) acknowledges the importance of clinicians developing trusting relationships with the communities we work with and serve. However, we would add that for true health equity, the Roles and Responsibilities Competency should include not only our roles to assess and address, but also *to partner* with communities to "advance the health of populations" (p. 10). Indeed, over 20 years ago, Drevdahl et al. (2001), in citing the 1998 Pew Health Professions Commission's Report which had called for health professionals to "embrace a personal ethic of social responsibility and service" (p. 28), further argued that nurses needed to develop "political competency" in order to more effectively advocate for policies that promote health equity and social justice (p. 29).

Dos and Don'ts for Community Advocacy

- Do your homework: Find out if anyone else or if another group in your organization is already working with the community. Be aware of your organization's reputation in the community-either good or bad; you may need to answer to it.
- Be mindful in framing your work: It is not about rescuing or being the savior or our agendas.
- Instead of a deficit model, use a strengths-based approach such as inclusive excellence and a focus on recognizing the importance of the local community's knowledge and capacity for self-advocacy and equitable partnerships.
- Trust takes time. Try to find an ally who can help break the ice and/or vouch for you.
- Be mindful of both your verbal and nonverbal communication and be intentional. There is a balance between offering to share your gifts and expertise versus being humble in the role as the learner of what the community defines as their wants and needs and the strengths they bring.

MACROSYSTEM

- Join/attend/present at interprofessional conferences such as the Society of Behavioral Medicine (www.sbm.org/about) or the American Interprofessional Health Collaborative (https://aihc-us.org/what-is-aihc) and identify opportunities to collaborate with colleagues at a national level.

- Join one of the professional boards and help draft position statements on increasing funding for the Supplemental Nutrition Assistance Program (SNAP), urban Americans' access to farmers' markets, and the amount that the U.S. Department of Agriculture allocates subsidies to organic fruit and vegetable farming.
- Call on the American Association of Colleges of Nursing (AACN) to ensure that not only care coordination and telehealth, but also political literacy and community advocacy skills are considered critical nurse competencies. Encourage the curriculum development of social determinants of health courses that medicine now has in 80% of its schools (American Association of Medical College, n.d.). Follow the advice of Kagan et al. (2014) and create an emancipatory nursing praxis that promotes both health and social justice. Also petition to require the National Council of State Boards of Nursing (NCSBN) to test for these competencies for nursing's prelicensure NCLEX exam.
- Call for policy changes to the Centers for Medicare & Medicaid Services (CMS) payment process for healthcare services; that is, policies that replace our downstream, fragmented health system with upstream models that can seamlessly support clients along the continuum of care. In order to have the power needed to change the entrenched care models, nurses will need to work collectively with their health systems and community service providers to advocate for funding for care coordination models and payment structures for the programs that improve client health self-management.
- Consider joining Lauren Underwood, Cori Bush, and other politician nurses by running for public office. Larson (2017) offers some excellent advice for nurses who wish to advocate for change by running for public office.

WHAT HAPPENS WHEN NURSES DON'T SPEAK UP AND BE PART OF THE SOLUTION

Despite increased national attention to the high maternal mortality rate, the numbers continue to climb. How has nursing science produced such a large body of effective health interventions, and yet so few of these interventions have been scaled up in our health system? For example, what is striking about the 2021 *MedPage Today's* (MPT; D'Ambrosio, 2021) article on maternal mortality *is not* the call for policy change but the lack of nursing consultation. Despite the accredited news service's commitment to educating *all* healthcare professionals, only physicians and their opinions about "medical services" and the responsibility of the "medical community" to improve pregnancy and postpartum care were consulted.

This piece specifically failed to mention how nursing interventions have made a difference. For example, the Nurse Family Partnership (NFP) has reduced maternal/child mortality through its program in which registered nurses follow Medicaid mothers prenatally through the first 2 years of the child's life (NFP, n.d.). Nurses can help Congress better understand the large return on investment if they were to partner with states to expand the NFP to all Medicaid-eligible women. Start by writing your congressional representatives, the ANA, and our other professional organizations and sharing the following Medicaid and Children's Health Insurance Program (CHIP) Payment and Access Commission (2020) statistics:

- Approximately 43% of all births in the United States were covered by Medicaid
- Among non-Hispanic women, Black women were more than twice as likely to be covered by Medicaid than White women (66% of births vs. 31%)
- Black women were half as likely as White women to have private health insurance (28% vs. 63%)

We could then ask for increased funding for the NFP which has over 40 years of evidence for not only improving maternal child birth outcomes but life trajectories (NFP, n.d.).

On the NFP website, you can also learn more about their work as well as ways to "take action" (NFP, 2021).

Learn about your local hospital's community health needs assessments (CHNA) and your community's prioritized health needs, and help figure out the barriers and facilitators to lasting change. For example, the DC Health Matters (2019) focuses on the same four areas (mental health, care coordination, health literacy, place-based care) as their 2016 report. Why do these problems persist, and how could new models of nursing care help solve them?

CASE STUDY: YOUR OWN COMMUNITY

A requirement of the Affordable Care Act is that all nonprofit hospitals conduct a community health needs assessment (CHNA) every 3 years. The American Hospital Association's (AHA) Community Health Improvement (AHA, n.d.) website provides an excellent overview and toolkit on creating/updating your local CHNA.

- Compare and contrast the priorities in the DC CHNA with your community's needs.

- Examine the organizations involved in your CHNA: congressional budget offices, health systems, government agencies, and so on.
- Ask yourself:
  - Do you know anyone who works for one of these agency partners?
  - Who could you contact to learn more about how you can help?
  - Are you a member of a Black church and/or have friends who are members?
- Once you have identified a community partner, collaborate with a community task force that can collectively identify and prioritize both program and policy goals.
  - What types of educational programs could be offered such as topics on health, political, and policing literacy?
  - A next step would developing a collective plan of action for creating sustainable change.
  - Encourage your community leaders and organizations to use Race Forward's (n.d.) toolkit to create a more equitable locality (www.raceforward.org/practice/tools/racial-equity-impact-assessment-toolkit).

CONCLUSION

This book focuses on developing the knowledge, attitudes, and skills needed to build an antiracism nursing practice. But we also need to focus on how to develop the skills to engage in action. A recent study by Motzkus et al. (2019) found a significant number of preclinical medical students endorsed recognizing implicit bias (84%) and practitioner self-reflection (74%), but only a small minority endorsed some form of action (22%), discussion (21%), or advocacy (18%). So how do we help future clinicians move beyond simply possessing the knowledge and attitudes and toward mastering the skills and behaviors of a clinician-citizen? We commit to being part of the solution by joining other health professions colleagues and scientists (Coulehan et al., 2003; Gruen et al., 2004) in becoming clinician-citizens.

The role of the nurse-citizen is to look beyond our practice and fight for health and social justice in the age of the COVID-19 pandemic. Using our structural competency framework, we must critically examine current policies that contribute to and/or exacerbate health disparities, as well as use our evidence-based practice skills to evaluate alternative models of care and identify which might best address and/or promote health equity.

Being a Nurse-Citizen

Being a nurse-citizen means that as clinicians we look beyond the healthcare system and the delivery of care and work collectively with our fellow citizen advocates and agents of change. Nurse-citizens need to critically examine the structural barriers to building trusting relationships with our clients. For example, what happens when we screen for vulnerabilities, but then don't have payment structures in place (e.g., the time and reimbursement rates) to develop an effective treatment plan that will holistically address our clients' health and well-being? We need to ask ourselves and our institutions what are we doing to ensure that we do more than just "treat'em and street'em" and truly establish effective care coordination.

We should also move beyond health equity to more broadly examine "equity and social justice." There are nearly 4 million nurses in the United States, so we have an opportunity to educate nurses on their ethical duty to participate in civic engagement and social dialogue about longstanding injustice in our communities. We need to think about our clients and communities more holistically and partner with other community service providers to promote equity, health, and well-being. We need to advocate for a paradigm change in healthcare that focuses on the holism of a person's life and not just when they enter the healthcare system. The Centers for Disease Control and Prevention (n.d.) offers an excellent resource center for clinicians to learn about and foster the movement toward "Health in All Policies." The time is now for each of us to become a nurse-citizen and help truly create a more *healthy and just* America.

REFERENCES

Acosta, K. L. (2020). Racism: A public health crisis. *City & Community, 19*(3), 506–515. https://doi.org/10.1111/cico.12518, https://onlinelibrary.wiley.com/doi/pdf/10.1111/cico.12518

American Association of Medical Colleges. (n.d.). Curriculum reports: Social determinants for health by academic level. https://www.aamc.org/data-reports/curriculum-reports/interactive-data/social-determinants-health-academic-level

American Hospital Association. (n.d.). Community health assessment toolkit. https://www.healthycommunities.org/resources/community-health-assessment-toolkit

American Nurses Association. (2020). ANA's membership assembly adopts resolution on racial justice for communities of color. https://www.nursingworld.org/news/news-releases/2020/ana-calls-for-racial-justice-for-communities-of-color/

Arao, B., & Clemens, K. (2013). From safe spaces to brave spaces. In *The art of effective facilitation: Reflections from social justice educators* (pp. 135–150). Stylus Publishing. https://culturallyresponsiveleadership.com/wp-content/uploads/2019/09/From-Safe-Spaces-to-Brave-Spaces.pdf

Baldwin, J. (2007/1972). *No name in the street: To be baptized* (pp. 404–474). Vintage.

Bevis, E. O. (1989). *Curriculum building in nursing: A process.* Jones & Bartlett Learning.

Bronfenbrenner, U. (1977). Toward an experimental ecology of human development. *American Psychologist, 32*(7), 513–531. https://doi.org/10.1037/0003-066X.32.7.513

Brusie, C. (2021, January 18). ANA president encourages nurses to get into politics and advocacy. https://nurse.org/articles/american-nurses-association-politics-advocacy/

Butler, S. M., Grabinsky, J., & Masi, D. (2015). *Hospitals as hubs to create healthy communities: Lessons from Washington Adventist Hospital.* The Brookings Institution. https://www.brookings.edu/wp-content/uploads/2016/07/Hospitals-as-Hubs-to-Create-Health-Communities.pdf

Centers for Disease Control and Prevention. (n.d.). Health in all policies. https://www.cdc.gov/policy/hiap/index.html

Clark, K., Miller, J., Leuning, C., & Baumgartner, K. (2017). The citizen nurse: An educational innovation for change. *Journal of Nursing Education, 56*(4), 247–250. https://doi.org/10.3928/01484834-20170323-12

Coulehan, J., Williams, P. C., McCrary, S. V., & Belling, C. (2003). The best lack all conviction: Biomedical ethics, professionalism, and social responsibility. *Cambridge Quarterly of Healthcare Ethics, 12*(1), 21–38.

D'Ambrosio, A. (2021, April 1). U.S. Maternal Mortality Rate climbs in 2019 – Despite national attention, racial disparities remain vast. *Medpage Today.* https://www.medpagetoday.com/obgyn/pregnancy/91888?xid=nl_mpt_SROBGYN_2021-04-03&eun=g435746d0r&utm_source=Sailthru&utm_medium=email&utm_campaign=ObGynUpdate_040321&utm_term=NL_Spec_OBGYN_Update_Active

DC Health Matters. (2019). Creating a culture of health. https://www.dchealthmatters.org/content/sites/washingtondc/DCHCC_CHIP_2017-2019_final_1.pdf

Drevdahl, D., Kneipp, S. M., Canales, M. K., & Dorcy, K. S. (2001). Reinvesting in social justice: A capital idea for public health nursing? *Advances in Nursing Science, 24*(2), 19–31.

Fairfax County Government. (n.d.). Opportunity neighborhoods practices guide. https://www.fairfaxcounty.gov/neighborhood-community-services/sites/neighborhood-community-services/files/assets/documents/prevention/opportunity%20neighborhood/opportunity%20neighborhood%20practices%20guide.pdf

Faulkner, D. (1949). Nurses are citizens. *American Journal of Nursing, 49*(1), 25–26.

Franklin, J. H., & The Advisory Board to the President's Initiative on Race. (1998, September). One America in the 21st century: Forging a new future: The President's initiative on race: The Advisory Board's report to the President. https://www.ncjrs.gov/txtfiles/173431.txt

Gailani, M. (2020, August 11). "Lifting as we climb" Mary Church Terrell and the 19th Amendment. https://tnmuseum.org/junior-curators/posts/lifting-as-we-climb-mary-church-terrell-and-the-19th-amendment

Garza, A. (2020, October 20). Black lives matter co-founder Alicia Garza on her book & creating change (Full stream interview 10/20). *Washington Post Live*. https://www.youtube.com/watch?v=nqDpH9zL5FA

Gatrall, C. E. (2020, October 29). Marie Branch and the power of nursing. https://nursingclio.org/2020/10/29/marie-branch-and-the-power-of-nursing/

Gonzalez, C. M., Deno, M. L., Kintzer, E., Marantz, P. R., Lypson, M. L., & McKee, M. D. (2019). A qualitative study of New York medical student views on implicit bias instruction: Implications for curriculum development. *Journal of General Internal Medicine, 34*(5), 692–698.

Grain, K. M., & Land, D. E. (2017). The social justice turn: Cultivating critical hope in an age of despair. *Michigan Journal of Community Service Learning, 23*(1).

Gruen, R. L., Pearson, S. D., & Brennan, T. A. (2004). Physician-citizens – Public roles and professional obligations. *JAMA, 291*(1), 94–98.

Hardy, B. (2020, November 16). Cori Bush, a nurse and activist, becomes the first Black woman to represent Missouri in Congress. *The New Yorker*. https://www.newyorker.com/magazine/2020/11/16/cori-bush-becomes-first-black-woman-and-first-nurse-to-represent-missouri-in-congress

Hill, C. (2020, December 28). Time magazine features Philly school nurse. https://www.phillytrib.com/news/local_news/time-magazine-features-philly-school-nurse/article_93de749f-5d81-55ca-9203-77e0116d2179.html

Interprofessional Education Collaborative. (2016). *Core competencies for interprofessional collaborative practice: 2016 update* (pp. 1–22). Author. https://hsc.unm.edu/ipe/resources/ipec-2016-core-competencies.pdf

Jones, M. M. (1949). Nurse-citizen in New England. *American Journal of Nursing, 49*(10), 616–617.

Kagan, P. N., Smith, M. C., & Chinn, P. L. (Eds.). (2014). *Philosophies and practices of emancipatory nursing: Social justice as praxis*. Routledge.

Krisberg, K. (2019). Programs work from within to prevent black maternal deaths: Workers targeting root cause-racism. *Nation's Health, 49*(6), 1–17.

Langer, E. (2011, August 18). Obituaries: Hazel Johnson-Brown Army nurse who was first black female general, dies at 83. https://www.washingtonpost.com/local/obituaries/hazel-johnson-brown-pioneering-black-army-nurse-dies-at-83/2011/08/18/gIQA0E2MOJ_story.html

Larson, J. (2017, June 5). Nurse legislators: Representing health care in state government. https://www.americanmobile.com/nursezone/nursing-news/nurse-legislators-representing-health-care-in-state-government/

Manton, A. (2016). Emergency nurse as citizen: The power of political action. *Journal of Emergency Nursing, 42*(5), 373–374.

Mason, D. J., Dickson, E., McLemore, M. R., & Pewrez, G. A. (2020). Frameworks for action in policy and politics. *Policy & Politics in Nursing and Health Care,* 1–16.

McNair, T. B., Bensimon, E. M., & Malcom-Piqueux, L. (2020). *From equity talk to equity walk: Expanding practitioner knowledge for racial justice in higher education.* John Wiley & Sons.

Medicaid and CHIP Payment and Access Commission. (2020). Financing maternity care: Medicaid's role. https://www.macpac.gov/wp-content/uploads/2020/01/Medicaid%E2%80%99s-Role-in-Financing-Maternity-Care.pdf

Merton, T. (1969). *My argument with the gestapo.* New Directions.

Mitchell, T. D. (2008). Traditional vs. critical service-learning: Engaging the literature to differentiate two models. *Michigan Journal of Community Service Learning, 14*(2), 50–65.

Momnibus. (n.d.). Black maternal health momnibus. https://blackmaternalhealthcaucus-underwood.house.gov/Momnibus

Motzkus, C., Wells, R. J., Wang, X., Chimienti, S., Plummer, D., Sabin, J., Allison, J., & Cashman, S. (2019). Pre-clinical medical student reflections on implicit bias: Implications for learning and teaching. *Plos One*, *14*(11), e0225058.

National League for Nursing. (2022). Beverly Malone. https://www.nln.org/about/staff/aboutwhos-who-at-the-nlnmanagement-team-bios/beverly-malone-0c9cb45c-7836-6c70-9642-ff00005f0421

National Trust. (n.d.). How Florence Nightingale influenced workhouse nursing. https://www.nationaltrust.org.uk/the-workhouse-southwell/features/how-florence-nightingale-influenced-workhouse-nursing

Nurse Family Partnership. (n.d.). Reductions in maternal and child mortality. https://www.nursefamilypartnership.org/about/proven-results/reductions-in-maternal-and-child-mortality/

Nurse Family Partnership. (2021). Take action. https://www.nursefamilypartnership.org/public-policy-and-advocacy/3take-action/

Office of the Governor of the Commonwealth of Virginia. (2021). ONE Virginia: Strategic plan for inclusive excellence: Measurement for change. https://www.governor.virginia.gov/media/governorvirginiagov/governor-of-virginia/pdf/toolkits/Measurement-for-Change-Presentation.pdf

Prevention Institute. (n.d.). Focus areas: Health equity and racial justice. https://www.preventioninstitute.org/focus-areas/health-equity-and-racial-justice

Race Forward. (n.d.). Racial equity impact assessment toolkit. https://www.raceforward.org/practice/tools/racial-equity-impact-assessment-toolkit

Seed The Way. (n.d.). Interrupting bias: Calling in vs. calling out. http://racialequityvtnea.org/educator-resources/appropriate-responses-to-injustice/

Staten, C. (2011, March 31). Mabel Keaton Staupers (1890–1989). *BlackPast.* https://www.blackpast.org/african-american-history/staupers-mabel-keaton-1890-1989/

Stone, S., Saucer, C., Bailey, M., Garba, R., Hurst, A., Jackson, S. M., Krueger, N., & Cokley, K. (2018). Learning while Black: A culturally informed model of the impostor phenomenon for Black graduate students. *Journal of Black Psychology, 44*(6), 491–531. https://doi.org/10.1177/0095798418786648

Thomas, G. R., Kaiser, B. L., & Svabek, K. (2017). The power of the personal: Breaking down stereotypes and building human connections. *Narrative Inquiry in Bioethics, 7*(1), 27–30. https://doi.org/10.1353/nib.2017.0010

Walker, A. (n.d.). Alice Walker: Beauty in truth. http://www.alicewalkerfilm.com/

Wisconsin Center for Nursing. (n.d.). Mary Elizabeth Mahoney – First African-American nurse. https://wicenterfornursing.org/mary-elizabeth-mahoney-first-african-american-nurse/

Yearby, R. (2020). *Racism is a public health crisis* [Doctoral dissertation, Saint Louis University]. https://ihje.org/wp-content/uploads/2020/12/Racism-is-a-Public-Health-Crisis.pdf

12

Multimedia Antiracism Toolkit

"Artists are the Gatekeepers of Truth."

—Paul Robeson (as cited by Sankofa.org)

We have compiled a list of resources including articles, songs, videos, and movies to inspire personal reflection, as well as start a dialogue in your practice, educational settings, and/or community group settings. Resources can be used alone and/or as enrichment to complement chapter readings.

In addition, we have created our own "Inclusive Excellence" playlist on Spotify that includes some of the songs in this toolkit as well as songs to inspire our work for change: https://open.spotify.com/playlist/0zCTMEEdgTq3k0FcaSAp3N?si=KBAA8KJ1TwKwY3ro4LCWXQ&dl_branch=1

We hope you enjoy these resources as much as we have.

The Learner Outcomes below can be achieved alone, with colleagues at work, and/or with friends, family members, and community groups.

- Start by sharing with each other your reactions to the piece; for example, hope, sadness, anger, frustration.
- Reflect on the historical context of the piece and then how it relates to the past, present, and future.
- What are key lessons learned?
- Explore how a particular resource helps ignite and inspire a desire to take action.

GROUP DIALOGUE RESOURCES

- **Structural Competency (n.d.):** https://structuralcompetency.org/training-materials
    - A resource website created by a transdisciplinary group of scholars and clinicians that provides training materials (including publications and past webinars) on the structural competency framework.
    - **Intersectionality Self Study Guide**: https://students.wustl.edu/intersectionality-self-study-guide/
    - Franklin, J. H. and the Advisory Board to the President's Initiative on Race. (1998, September). ***One America in the 21st century: Forging a new future: The President's initiative on race: The Advisory Board's report to the President.*** https://www.ncjrs.gov/txtfiles/173431.txt
        - A step-by-step guide for organizations and community groups on how individuals, community groups, and/or organizations can come together to talk about race.
        - Even after 20 years, the format and questions are timely and relevant to America's dialogue on race.

Breaking Down Barriers: National Geographic Society's (n.d.) 10-minute video https://www.nationalgeographic.org/video/breaking-down-barriers/

- Compare and contrast the conversations between Tara and Kenya at the beginning and then at the end of the video. Notice both the verbal and nonverbal communication.
- How does Tara include Colin as a way to defend herself? What do the others do in response?
- What do you think led to the change and how do you think each of them changed?
- How does this video help us reflect on our own reactions during conversations around race?

The Circle Way: http://www.thecircleway.net/the-circle-way

- Learn about the process for conducting a "circle way" gathering.
- How might this process help to increase inclusion and opportunity for new voices/perspectives to be shared?

POETRY

Amanda Gorman's "The Hill We Climb"
https://www.youtube.com/watch?v=LZ055ilIiN4

- Teaching "The Hill We Climb"
  - https://www.tolerance.org/magazine/teach-this-the-hill-we-climb-and-the-2021-inauguration
- Michelle Obama interviews Amanda Gorman for *Time* Magazine, February 4, 2021
  - https://time.com/5933596/amanda-gorman-michelle-obama-interview/

Maya Angelou's Poem "On the Pulse of Morning"
https://www.youtube.com/watch?v=59xGmHzxtZ4

- Compare and contrast the two poems by Ms. Angelou and Ms. Gorman and how they are situated within their respective historical context?
- How do they each inspire hope?
- Do you think their age and/or personal lived experiences are expressed or are they speaking for all?
- For additional insights on Ms. Angelou's work, consider watching the episode from the Iconoclast Series: Dave Chappelle + Maya Angelou:
- https://www.youtube.com/watch?v=okc6COsgzoE

Lokela Blanc "Black and white America: a Sunday Poem" (February 14, 2021)
http://art19.com/shows/5-things/episodes/176408b9-1f68-49ce-9cfb-26cb5edb4020

- 15-minute podcast where Saint-Lucian/Haitian journalist, Lokela Blanc, discusses her recently published poem, "blak and (h)wit" and her struggles in both predominately Black and predominately White spaces.
- Particularly poignant is her realization that it was her interactions with the White people that she learned about her blackness.

Let America be America Again by Langston Hughes

https://www.poetryfoundation.org/poems/147907/let-america-be-america-again

- How do you feel about the America Mr. Hughes describes? How does it contrast with the other selected poems here?
- Do you agree it has not been the dream so many Americans thought it would be? Why or why not?
- What is his hope for this country?
- In what ways is he trying to unify the country?

LITERATURE (BOOKS, ARTICLES)

Women, Race, and Memory: An Excerpt From Toni Morrison's New Book, The Source of Self-Regard

https://theattic.jezebel.com/women-race-and-memory-an-excerpt-from-toni-morrisons-1832540444

- What do you think about Morrison's assertion, "Complicity in the subjugation of race and class accounts for much of the self-sabotage women are prey to..."?
  - How does her opening and closing of the essay on Harriet Tubman's story strengthen her arguments?
- Companion article by Biana, H.T. (2020) "Extending Bell Hooks' Feminist Theory" https://vc.bridgew.edu/cgi/viewcontent.cgi?article=2207&context=jiws
- There is 30 years distance between Morrison's and Biana's essays: What has changed and what has not?
- Where do we go from here? How might building alliances across, class, race, and gender help bring about equity and justice?
- For a deeper examination, watch: **Toni Morrison: The Pieces I Am (2020)** https://www.pbs.org/wnet/americanmasters/toni-morrison-the-pieces-i-am-documentary/16971/

Time's Witness by Michael Malone (1983)

- What did you think about Police Chief Mangum's beliefs about race, class, and injustice?
- How does the intersectionality of his own life (redneck, Vietnam veteran, police officer, and PhD candidate) impact his personal and professional relationships?
- **Were you surprised by Judge Roche's sentence for the young Black rioters?**

- **Do you agree with her that jail is "incredibly expensive, largely ineffective, and usually inhumane"?**
- How did her sentence help promote healing and opportunity for the community?

Noel Ignatiev's Long Fight Against Whiteness

https://www.newyorker.com/news/postscript/noel-ignatievs-long-fight-against-whiteness

- Kang's (2019) tribute to Dr. Ignatiev's work includes an overview of his book, *How the Irish Became White* and his life of activism to move our society beyond racial division.
- What do you think about Ignatiev's concept about the Civil War inside the White mind: Where Whites believe they should side with their White bosses and leaders over solidarity with their fellow Black, Indigenous, and People of Color (BIPOCs) who are stuck in a rigged economic paradigm?
- How have your life experiences informed your reaction to his premise?

What a Real President was Like – Bill Moyers (1988)

https://www.washingtonpost.com/archive/opinions/1988/11/13/what-a-real-president-was-like/d483c1be-d0da-43b7-bde6-04e10106ff6c/?utm_term=.bacafc2e3795

- What was your reaction to President Johnson's assessment of the racial epithets he saw on signs while traveling in the South? Do you believe the explanation is still true today?
- How did President Johnson's beliefs and actions improve the lives of Black America?
- Twenty years later, how had the lives of America's most vulnerable improved?

Men We Reaped **by Jesmyn Ward and** ***A Promised Land*** **by Barack Obama**

- Compare and contrast the lived experiences of these two authors.
- Ward captures the intersectionality of Black men growing up in the rural South. She also helps us to better understand the phenomenon of "internalized racism."
  - https://www.youtube.com/watch?v=xgLKWjhwhkk
- Ward's interview with President Obama for his book, *The Promised Land* (November, 2020)
  - https://www.vanityfair.com/style/2020/11/barack-obama-jesmyn-ward-interview

- Were you surprised by President Obama's discussion about what can unite us even if we have such diverse lived experiences?
    - *Vanity Fair* (2020). Power to tell the story; *Vanity Fair* (2020) Breonna Taylor and guest-editor: The noticeable difference when there is intentional inclusion and giving voice to Black Culture. https://archive.vanityfair.com/issue/20200901

Critical Race Theory

Article: *"I See My Work as Talking Back": How Critical Race Theory Mastermind Kimberlé Crenshaw Is Weathering the Culture Wars*

https://www.vanityfair.com/news/2021/07/how-critical-race-theory-mastermind-kimberle-crenshaw-is-weathering-the-culture-wars

- How did this article help you to better understand Critical Race Theory?
- How did it compare to what you have heard or seen in the media?
- How would you like to see Critical Race Theory incorporated into nursing curricula?

Environmental Justice

Read: Bullard, R. D. (2001). Environmental justice in the 21st century: Race still matters. *Phylon, 49*(3/4), 151–171. Downloaded from: http://majorsmatter.net/race/Readings/Bullard%202001.pdf

- Reflect on your understanding of the history of the United States Environmental Justice Movement.
- What were your reactions to the sobering discussion on the institutional racism which argues that "corporate welfare to polluters" and "lax enforcement of environmental regulations" have come at the expense of citizen health?

Listen to the Podcast or Read the Transcript: *How the Pandemic Changed Us:* https://revealnews.org/episodes/how-the-pandemic-changed-us/

- Reflect on the Dr. Sacoby Wilson's assertion that White supremacy decides "who is able to access clean air and clean water and who's not."
- Discuss the impact that local, state, and federal policies have on environmental justice and health equity.

Dear Mrs. L'Engle. Santamaria, A. (March 2021). https://archive.vanityfair.com/article/2021/3/dear-mrs-lengle

- Tells the story of famed author, Madeleine L'Engle, and incarcerated person, Ahmad Rahman, who were part of the PEN America Writing Award for Prisoners.
- Were you surprised by their unlikely friendship?
- What other social supports and opportunities helped Dr. Rahman achieve his professional dream?
- How did Dr. Rahman's life experiences impact his work with the next generation of aspiring youth?

VIDEOS

Historic debate between William F. Buckley and James Baldwin at Cambridge University (1965)

https://www.youtube.com/watch?v=oFeoS41xe7w

- A powerful moment when Baldwin notes, "the disaffection and demoralization" that occurs when a young Black child realizes that in this "glittering republic" of their birth there is not "any place for you." (minutes: 18:22–19:21).
  - Consider the fact that over 50 years later we still have the American policing problem that is referenced by Mr. Baldwin. Is this what Mr. Buckley meant when he said, "there is no instant cure for the race problem in America"? (minute 49:14).

James Baldwin on the Black Experience in America (In 1960 interviewed by Canadian Nathan Cohen) (8:04 minutes)

- The tensions between the races is not a southern problem, but a national problem that began after the Civil War.

TED-Ed: *Notes of a native son: The world according to James Baldwin* (Christina Greer, February 2019). (4:13 minutes) https://www.youtube.com/watch?v=dKku0AfTs0c

- "People are trapped in history and history is trapped in them." (minute 2:44)
- Do you agree with Baldwin that racism hurts both Whites and Blacks?
- For additional learning see 35 curated quotes in *The Oprah Magazine* https://www.oprahmag.com/life/g32842156/james-baldwin-quotes/?slide=7

Locker, M. (August 19, 2019). John Oliver, Larry David, and Wanda Sykes Give Medical Bias the "Last Week Tonight" Treatment

- Ms. Locker provides an excellent summary and link to the *Last Week with John Oliver* episode

- John Oliver teams up with Larry David and Wanda Sykes to talk about bias in healthcare: https://money.yahoo.com/john-oliver-larry-david-wanda-091224904.html?guccounter=1&guce_referrer=aHR0cHM6Ly93d3cuZ29vZ2xlLmNvbS8&guce_referrer_sig=AQAAAIGyoimBPaQyLhU74I7hZE6cSePyru7j0oSFv-bqXBKd42khU-nVoHsL56lmAnRdhbGo7dPeEzz5TNRdZWaxwvQ0odpE6D6vUMSOsUfs8QmnDtQ-ng6rVKyg-rFz2JrZx6fyuL3w0raobq2CQOLh2AvuCbqKPnlnpgjz5TGCpu8g
- What do you think about Wanda Sykes' four recommendations?
- In what ways does her comedic stance make her message more effective?

Black Panthers White Lies: Dr. Curtis Austin, TEDxOhioStateUniversity: https://www.youtube.com/watch?v=KPN8LHVeFYA

- Did you think it was possible in the 21st century that a university professor could be wrongly charged by the FBI?
- What did you know about the Black Panther Party before this talk?
- How does his invitation for us to do our own research increase the credibility of his position?
- How does his plea for inclusivity for the cause make you feel?
- What was your reaction at the end when he raised his hand and concluded with "So I say to you power to the people"?

Dupre, K. (12 October, 2016). **Black is not a weapon.** https://mashable.com/article/against-the-wall-police-violence-film#3o9NHLElamqF

- Public service announcement (PSA) commissioned for Sankofa.org
- Why did Director-Partners Bush and Renz use Black celebrities and activists to make their PSA "Against the Wall"?
- How do the real-life 911 tapes and newscasts help to "resensitize" us to persistent and pervasive police brutality against the Black community?
- Do you agree with the narrator that this isn't an "accident" but a "message" being sent?

Daryl Davis (December 8, 2017) Why I, as a Black man, attend KKK rallies

https://www.youtube.com/watch?v=ORp3q1Oaezw

- Accomplished musician and actor who delivers an inspiring TEDxNaperville talk about his experiences of racism growing up and living in America.

- Describes his journey in trying to understand hate from reading books to meeting with those who hate.
- What inspires you most about his story?

UNCF (1977) "A Mind Is a Terrible Thing to Waste" (video)

- https://www.youtube.com/watch?v=9UcnABDsGbo
- What are some of the positive messaging seen as far as education and professional opportunities?
- Is there a difference between how men and women are portrayed?
- Who are the majority of "power brokers" in the commercial?

***Henrietta Lacks' "Immortal" Impact on Research Now Extends to Patient Consent*;** PBS Newshour (August 8, 2013)

https://www.pbs.org/newshour/show/henrietta-lacks-immortal-impact-on-medical-research

- How did race factor into the decisions that researchers made with Henrietta Lacks's cell line?
- How will this story impact your clinical practice?

Video: *The Death of Emmett Till*: https://www.history.com/this-day-in-history/the-death-of-emmett-till Along with its companion link, it reminds us that Emmett Till's death was 8 years to the date that Dr. Martin Luther delivered his "I Have A Dream" speech: https://www.history.com/news/same-date-8-years-apart-from-emmett-till-to-i-have-a-dream-in-photos

- We have friends, family members, and fellow Americans who were alive when Emmett Till was murdered and Dr. King gave his speech. Reflecting on the "chronos" of their lives, what effect might that have on their perceptions and feelings around race in America?

Cultural Humility Video by Vivian Chavez (2012) https://www.youtube.com/watch?v=SaSHLbS1V4w

- Interviews with Drs. Tervalon and Murray-Garcia about the genesis of their 1998 article on cultural humility.
- Why was there a need to move from "competency" to "humility"?
- Are you still hearing the term "competency" or "sensitivity" in your professional circles?
  - Why do you think that we are still hearing these terms after more than 20 years?
  - In what ways does cultural humility help us more effectively address structural racism?

PODCASTS /MOVIES/TV SHOWS

Panel 1: Kenya Beard – Future of Nursing 2030 Seattle Town Hall: High Tech to High Touch
https://www.youtube.com/watch?v=xFOyteIux60

- Dr. Beard shares her grandfather's feelings about unequal care. The Landmark Institute of Medicine study came out over 20 years ago, so why do you think disparities still persist?
- Technology such as computer tablets to help with translation services can help promote health equity, but as Dr. Beard points out, they can also harm. How does your practice use technology and what can you do to reduce the risk of harm to your clients?
- Dr. Beard, highlights the paradox for nurses: "The nursing profession, we are rooted in social justice, however, we live in a socially unjust world." What can you do individually, and then collectively with your colleagues and communities to help promote health equity, and places of inclusion and belonging?
- How can nurses take their knowledge of social determinants of health and advocate for policies that truly address the racism in healthcare and governmental policies?

Second Episode of Renegades: Born in the USA. (February 19, 2021). A Spotify Podcast by President Obama and Bruce Springsteen: https://open.spotify.com/episode/3ba69iXo04u9XoRsHsX9N0

- Compare and contrast their experiences with race in America.
- Reflect on how "racism" gets under the skin and President Obama's statement about the "cuts" that come from the unexpected and heartbreaking moments when the race card is played.
- How does their conversation help others have the courage to talk about race?

Podcast Series: **Code Sw!tch Race. In Your Face.**
https://www.npr.org/sections/codeswitch/

- Topics include: The Tulsa massacre, voting rights issues, and the catalyzing effect of George Floyd's death for racial reckoning both nationally and internationally.
- Listen alone or in a group and then share reflections, feelings, and ideas for change.

Spike Lee's Blackkklansman (2018) https://www.youtube.com/watch?v=pFc6I0rgmgY

- **(August 10, 2018) Julie Miller compares and contrasts the movie with the real-life experiences of Officer Ron**

Stallworth. https://www.vanityfair.com/hollywood/2018/08/blackkklansman-ron-stallworth-true-story-spike-lee-kkk

- **(February 25, 2021) Matthew Dessum** https://slate.com/culture/2021/02/judas-black-messiah-true-story-fred-hampton-accuracy.html
- What do you think about movies that change important details in a person's story? Does it help with creating interest or does it reduce its credibility?

Antebellum (18 September, 2020) https://www.phillytrib.com/entertainment/movies/antebellum-is-a-nightmare-come-true-for-writer-gerard-bush/article_d6f995b4-0146-54fe-9bb7-1cd0ad37cc21.html

- What is unique about this film compared to other films that portray the inhumanity of slavery?
- How does linking the present to the past amplify feelings of fear and horror?

The Black Church: This is our story. This is our song. https://www.pbs.org/show/black-church/

- Why is it so important for Americans to understand the history of the Black church?
- How has the song of the Black church influenced music in America?
- How does this knowledge help foster a strengths-based approach to addressing inequality?

Wake Up (scene from "black-ish") https://www.youtube.com/watch?v=VvykfyGTnbQ

- Compare and contrast the generational differences/similarities of the family members as they watch the news.
- How does the intersection of race, class, and gender present itself in the dialogue between the two parents?
- What parts of the scene most affected you and why?

MUSIC

John Mellencamp's Pink Houses (1983) Versus Our Country (2007)

- What was similar about the problems in America in 1983 versus 2007?
- How were Blacks and Whites portrayed in each of the videos?
- How do these two songs relate to Mr. Hughes's poem, "Let America Be America Again"?

Whitney Houston's radical reclamation of 'The Star Spangled Banner'

https://www.youtube.com/watch?v=N_lCmBvYMRs

- Read the Tensley's 2021 analysis of her performance and think about the public's perceptions then and now? Do you remember the performance and/or conversations about it?
  - https://www.cnn.com/2021/02/07/politics/whitney-houston-national-anthem-super-bowl-racial-justice/index.html
- TwinsthenewTrend Reaction to Whitney Houston's Superbowl performance (2020)
  - https://www.youtube.com/watch?v=TMOa-mqNmOY
  - How does seeing her performance through the "Twins'" eyes impact your feelings about the performance?

Tim McGraw and Beyonce both celebrate their Southern heritage in these two songs:

Beyonce's Formation https://www.youtube.com/watch?v=WDZJPJV__bQ

Tim McGraw's Southern Voice https://www.youtube.com/watch?v=RdT8Tlzto20

- Compare and contrast their messages about the South.
- How does Tim McGraw celebrate Black America?
- What does Beyonce say about White supremacy?

Two versions of a song that leads us to ask ourselves is it really, "The Way It Is"?

- Tupac "Changes" (1998): https://www.youtube.com/watch?v=eXvBjCO19QY
- Bruce Hornsby "The Way It Is" (1986): https://www.youtube.com/watch?v=cOeKidp-iWo
- Reflect on the words of "Changes" about the American presidency and race. Do you think America at that time believed that 10 years later it would be possible to elect the first Black president? Why or why not?

Compare and contrast these two country songs and how they portray Black, Indigenous, and People of Color (BIPOCs)

Blake Shelton's "Boys Round Here" https://www.youtube.com/watch?v=JXAgv665J14

- Think about how the video starts, what are the stereotypes about urban Black Americans and the White Americans?
- What do you think about the ending?
- Do you think it helps with racial understanding?

Tim McGraw's Humble and Kind https://www.youtube.com/watch?v=awzNHuGqoMc

- What is different about Tim McGraw's song?
- What language is inclusive and what language isn't?

How do these songs inspire hope for America today?

- **"Glory" Common and John Legend**
  - Celebrating the 1965 "Bloody Sunday" walk from Selma to Montgomery as part of the voting rights movement. https://www.youtube.com/watch?v=HUZOKvYcx_o
  - 55 years later, as our country has another racial reckoning, how does this song acknowledge the feelings of being tired, but still offer hope?

- **"Better Days" Ant Clemons and Justin Timberlake** https://www.youtube.com/watch?v=u4HkM6WzmFY
- **"Undivided" Tim McGraw and Tyler Hubbard** https://www.youtube.com/watch?v=nsFb67fo7nE
  - How does the message of compassion in this song help heal and unite folks?
  - How does judgment divide us?
  - What is being asked of each of us to make change?

Tenney. L. (2019) Being An Active Bystander
From the Kirwan Institute (Under "Final Thoughts" >> "Additional Resources") https://kirwaninstitute.osu.edu/sites/default/files/2019-08/Active_Bystander_Handout_2019.pdf

- Compare and contrast this tool with Seed The Way's (n.d.) "Interrupting Bias: Calling Out vs. Calling In" http://www.racialequityvtnea.org/wp-content/uploads/2018/09/Interrupting-Bias_-Calling-Out-vs.-Calling-In-REVISED-Aug-2018-1.pdf
- Why does context matter for the strategy you use as an active bystander?
- Start a group discussion with reflections on when colleagues have used one or the other. Examples:
  - Are there times you wished you had used a different strategy and if so, why?
  - Are there times when you wished someone else had used a different strategy to call you in versus call you out?

Health Disparities:

- **Toxic Stress**: https://developingchild.harvard.edu/science/key-concepts/toxic-stress/#:~:text=Toxic%20stress%20response%20 can%20occur,hardship%E2%80%94without%20adequate%20adult%20support.

- **The Entire "Unnatural Causes" 8-Part Series;** in particular:
- *When the Bough Breaks*: Full transcript—the high cost of racism and its effects on Black perinatal outcomes: https://unnaturalcauses.org/assets/uploads/file/UC_Transcript_2.pdf
- The series premiered in 2008 so what has and has not changed since then?
- Why is Syme's concept "Control of Destiny" so important to human health and well-being?
    - Use the Brofenbrenner model to frame a discussion on the barriers and facilitators to addressing inequality and health equity.

THE IMPORTANCE OF CHRIS ROCK'S COMEDY TO HELP US THINK DEEPLY

As you listen and watch Chris Rock, reflect on the quote below:

"The world is a comedy to those that think; a tragedy to those that feel."

– Horace Walpole (en.wikiquote.org)

- Chris Rock:The Importance of Inclusive Excellence

"Chris Rock on 'Top Five' comedy and race": Charlie Rose interviews Chris Rock about the movie he "wrote, directed, and starred." The movie, "Top Five," examines Black fame and the differences in pressure for White versus Black celebrities. https://www.youtube.com/watch?v=yyFGpJ9Hq2U

- What was your reaction to Chris Rock's explanation about why he prefers an all-Black audience when filming his HBO specials?
- Charlie Rose quotes that Seinfeld says, "Chris Rock can do race better than anyone…get to the truth of race in America." And then there's Chris Rock's response, "I really, really, really, really, know it." The fine line between tragedy and comedy…
- Rock, C. (December 3, 2014) "Chris Rock Pens Blistering Essay on Hollywood's Race Problem: 'It's a White Industry' Essay": https://www.hollywoodreporter.com/news/top-five-filmmaker-chris-rock-753223
- Interview with Gayle King (January 3, 2021) https://www.youtube.com/watch?v=Pt0TIwtpImo
- Candid interview—It's inspiring how he openly talks about his therapy and what matters.

- What was your reaction when he stated there are some professions (like pilots) where we cannot have bad apples? Should we hold our clinicians and police officers to the same zero tolerance for harm?
- The Chris Rock Show—Confederate Flag (June 2012)

https://www.youtube.com/watch?v=SZ8_49BRSiw

- How did the feelings about the flag differ across racial lines?
- How does Chris Rock use humor to tell both sides of the issue of South Carolina's Confederate battle flag?
- Caitlin Byrd (September 2020) looks back at what has changed 5 years after the flag's removal: https://www.postandcourier.com/politics/5-years-ago-south-carolina-brought-down-the-confederate-flag-it-was-just-the-beginning/article_62b7e0f6-bfc1-11ea-808f-6f165bc5ed6e.html
  - What was the catalyst for lawmakers to finally remove the flag?
  - According to those interviewed, was it helpful?
  - What has changed and not changed about systemic racism in the state?

Index

Index

www.ingramcontent.com/pod-product-compliance
Ingram Content Group UK Ltd.
Pitfield, Milton Keynes, MK11 3LW, UK
UKHW021103170926
15229UKWH00007B/23

9 780826 184528